WHAT THE BLEEP BRAIN?

Techniques to Train Your Brain, Reset your Nervous System, and Live a Better Life

Copyright © 2024 Todd Nyholm

All rights reserved. No part of this publication may be reproduced, distributed, or transmitted in any form or by any means, including photocopying, recording, or other electronic or mechanical methods, without the prior written permission of the publisher, except in the case of brief quotations embodied in critical reviews and certain other noncommercial uses permitted by copyright law. For permission

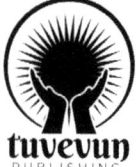

requests, write to the publisher, addressed "Attention: Permissions Coordinator," at the address below.

Tuvevun@gmail.com

ISBN: 978-1-7343734-2-4 (paperback)
ISBN: 978-1-7343734-3-1 (ebook)

Ordering Information:
Special discounts are available on quantity purchases by corporations, associations, and others. For details, contact Tuvevun@gmail.com

WHAT THE BLEEP BRAIN?

Techniques to Train Your Brain, Reset your Nervous System, and Live a Better Life

TODD NILS NYHOLM

TABLE OF CONTENTS

	Introduction	1
	This Book Is Written a Bit Differently	9
chapter 1	*Working with Your Hardware*	11
chapter 2	*Senses Meditation*	15
chapter 3	*How These Methods Came About and a History*	21
chapter 4	*Trauma Directly Affects Your Brain and Central Nervous System*	27
chapter 5	*Debugging Your Mental Software*	31
chapter 6	*The Power Breath*	41
chapter 7	*A Desperate Need*	47
chapter 8	*Cascade Meditation*	51
chapter 9	*Meditative States*	57
chapter 10	*Cascading Joint Meditations*	67
chapter 11	*The Why of Changing State (Reaching Your Inner World)*	71
chapter 12	*Attention*	75
chapter 13	*The Activating Methods*	81
chapter 14	*The Activating Methods*	91
chapter 15	*Personal Experience of the Full Method (What You Might Expect)*	101
chapter 16	*The Push Breath*	109
chapter 17	*Rewriting Your History*	113
chapter 18	*Set Two of the Activating Methods*	119
chapter 19	*"Mind Storm," Memory, and Anxiety*	127

chapter 20	*For a Better Life*	**131**
chapter 21	*The Meninges Meditation*	**137**
chapter 22	*The Empowered Breath Method*	**143**
chapter 23	*Why Is this Book Different from the First Two?*	**149**
chapter 24	*Occupy All of You*	**153**
chapter 25	*The Final Series of the Activating Methods*	**157**
chapter 26	*The Flow Meditation*	**161**
chapter 27	*Importance and Value of the Activating Methods*	**165**
chapter 28	*The Vital Brain Method*	**169**
chapter 29	*Final Thoughts*	**189**
chapter 30	*Glossary*	**191**
	Endnotes	**199**

> I really like doing the brain stuff. It feels good. It's like scratching the deepest itch. —**C. P.**

> The amount of change these methods have given me is astounding. It's made a huge difference in my life both physically and mentally. —**J. T.**

> I feel like my function has improved by 10%. My mind feels clearer and my emotions are calmer. I'm really surprised by the changes I've gotten. —**P. C.**

HERE IS A MIND MAP FOR ALL OF YOU WHO LIKE TO FLIP TO THE FRONT OF A BOOK TO SEE IF IT'S FOR YOU. I SEE YOU, YOU'RE MY PEOPLE. I DO THE SAME THING.

For self-development:

- Learn ways to gain better control of your nervous system.
- Develop a practice to gain control over your brain states.
- Develop tools to work on yourself inside.
- Learn to systematically upgrade your nervous system by working with it directly.
- Build a toolset for working with yourself.

For meditation:

- Meditation is often poorly understood and sometimes even feared. Explore methods to help you gain familiarity with your inner states.
- Learn methods for creating meditative states through an in-depth method that works with your anatomy.
- Learn methods for changing your inner state—how you feel and function through simple breathing exercises.
- Discover—through your own work—that a major part of meditation is recovering more of who you are inside.

For making consciousness and emotional changes:

- Gain understanding of how your breathing, your brain states, and your attention affect your emotions.
- Learn to reset your emotional thermostat through a method that helps to turn on aspects of your nervous system and turn them off again.

- Gain appreciation that your emotions are not random things that happen to you but are reflections of many things going on within you.
- Practice a method to use your emotions to improve your moment-to-moment experience.

For learning to work with the brain and brain states:

- Take more control of your inner state.
- Gain understanding of how your brainwaves affect your life experiences.
- Learn how to work with your brain to make your life better.
- Learn techniques to consciously make changes to your brain state.

For health development and to help people with chronic illness:

- Learn methods for building your overall health by working from the inside out.
- Work toward developing your sense of well-being—to actually feel good in your body right now.
- Learn a method that fundamentally helped the author recover from Lyme disease, fibromyalgia, chronic fatigue, and other health issues.
- Explore the relationship between the mind, emotions, and body, to understand how interconnected they are to your health and experience of life.

INTRODUCTION

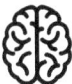

THIS BOOK IS WRITTEN FOR everyone who struggles with getting a handle on their inner world, which can be defined as including your mind, your emotions, the inner workings of your body, and the energy you bring to your life. Understanding and making the best use of these aspects of yourself requires a method—a path that you can work from.

Part of the problem for many of us is that we are so focused on our outer, tangible world that we miss what's going on inside us. Our inner world seems intangible—untouchable—within our bodies. And yet, this part of us actually *can* be touched. It is touched by our attention. We will talk about attention quite a bit in this book.

I have often stated in interviews and in my books that life is really experienced from within. You take information in, your nervous system builds a model for you of what is going on in the world, and then your hormones and neurotransmitters chemically create how you feel. The process of what happens inside you—both its tangible and intangible aspects—is what creates your life's experiences.

As a Somatic Therapist,[1] I have spent decades focused on wellness education and the connection between mind and body. In my search for an answer to the question of how to successfully live a healthy and vital life, I realized that it has to start with working with your inner world. I designed the systems of the Nytality Method[2] as a solution and a methodology to do just that and I can promise that they work brilliantly. Earlier in my life, I felt like I was struggling minute to minute due to health problems, past trauma, and seemingly unattainable personal aims. I now feel like I'm soaring inside—and I did it through my own efforts applying the principles of the Nytality Method. It is my passion to teach these systems to as many people as possible throughout the world.

Each of my books focuses on one of the 15 systems that make up the Nytality Method. The first was written to help readers understand what sabotages diet, weight, and health goals. The second provides principles to help guide you to conduct your life like a beautiful symphony. This book, the third in the series, takes those principles a step further, to help you get into your nervous system and work with it in a way that makes your life better.

The system described in this book can be used for self-development: helping you gain control over your inner workings. You will begin to make interesting changes in your brain states and learn how to give yourself a "nervous-system upgrade"—just like upgrading your computer— allowing you to function faster and with less resistance, pain, and confusion. As you will discover, it is a wonderful experience to find that your mind is moving faster, making better connections, and is no longer getting stuck in the past or the future. And it is life-changing to feel your emotions settle in and work with you in a direct way—think of the symphony I spoke of earlier. Your emotions are like an orchestra that you can direct, while at the same time, they are able to give you information about life and yourself.

In this book you will also learn about meditation and meditative states. Most people don't really understand meditation or how to do it; we will talk about that to help clarify the mystery. And I'll give you direct methods to create and experience meditative states and help you understand meditation's value in your daily life.

The chapters ahead will help you understand your brain states: how they affect your daily life and the ways in which you function—and not just in a theoretical way. I provide precise descriptions on how to achieve desirable brain states and information on the hows and whys of creating conscious control over them in your daily life.

For those of you struggling with chronic health issues, the system described in this book can provide hope as you confront the confusing abyss of methods and treatments for healing yourself. When you begin to upgrade your own system, all kinds of chronic situations begin to heal—seemingly of themselves. In reality, upgrading your system means removing the blockage from healthy functioning so your system is better able to regulate itself. For example, you might have struggled with sleep and now you sleep pleasantly like a baby. And because you can sleep and your body can adequately heal and rebuild, your fibromyalgia pain completely dissipates. This is not a theory, this happened to me.

For those of you without health issues, what if you could practice a method that helps you to maintain your health from the inside out long into your later years?

One of my core purposes in establishing this method was to find a way to turn the emotional system off and on again like rebooting a computer. How do you reset the emotional system so that it isn't stuck in the past? How do you guide it to function as a means toward achieving a higher level of flexible options for how your emotions work and how your nervous system regulates them? I want people who have experienced enough trauma in their lives to feel stuck to realize that it is possible not only to get unstuck but also to go way beyond that. You will always remember the trauma, but you don't need to be stuck.

How does the system in this book provide solutions to these problems?

Most people want to make their lives better in some noticeable way through their own efforts. This is what the Nytality Method can do for you.

The particular system outlined in this book, which I call the Vital Brain Method, tackles working with your central nervous system, using it to change your mental and emotional states to help you live a healthier, happier life. In doing so, you will be able to expand your consciousness.

Expansion of consciousness is difficult to explain because it's your own perception of what's in front of you that changes. Let me give a few hints about how that works. When your consciousness expands, you become less identified with your body, mind, and emotions. You experience separation between your consciousness and those parts of yourself.

For example, where previously you might have been pushed emotionally to scream at a bad driver, now you feel calm in a situation that would have created rage. Or perhaps you've never been able to get your thoughts—and particularly intrusive thoughts—to slow down. Now you have moments where your mind is clear, settled, and quiet. This really does change your experience of life in a beautiful way.

I've discovered over the years that most people are unwilling to make those kinds of changes to their thinking. I believe this is largely because they are unaware of their own blocks and the wonderful possibilities that are created when those blocks are removed. People have a surprising connection to suffering, attachment, and identification. They work hard to hold on to their suffering and will also work hard to justify it through their thoughts and actions.

You are much greater than you think you are, and you have extraordinary potential. Regardless of anything else about you—especially any outer characteristics that you think define you—your potential goes deeper than that. *You* are deeper than that. Hopefully, at least in part, you are reading this book because you think or feel that might be true.

The inner states you can create for yourself are full of interesting possibilities, and those states will radiate out into the rest of your life—including your outer life—changing it to be more of what you want. But these possibilities don't develop randomly. They have to be sought after, chased, wooed, developed, and ultimately worked for. Nothing will ask more of you, because it will take every part of you working together harmoniously to make it happen. Please don't make the mistake of thinking that I mean it has to hurt (perhaps some of it will, and that can be a wonderful experience); however, it will require consistency—practiced, uplifted, and synergistically directed—to encourage the change you desire to happen and to make it who and what you are.

But it is so beautiful, it's worth every drop of you that you put into it.

This book tells the story of how the Nytality Method came about, arising out of my intense need for its techniques. It also serves as a manual for how to get started in adopting the core of the method into your own life. It is built on the interconnected nature of how the human mind and body work. Assume that each part of you is doing more than you realize to connect with every other part of you.

You are in control of the state you are in. My method will help you to methodically build a staircase within yourself to expand your consciousness, step-by-step. Once you've reached the top, you'll never be able to see the world the same again. Your view has changed. Your mind has changed. Your emotions have changed. Even your body is different. Certainly, you experience it that way. These changes have opened up my consciousness in ways beyond anything I could have conceived. Now, I want to share them with you.

It would be hard for me to accurately convey the changes I've experienced in how I function mentally, emotionally, physically, and spiritually through following these methods. My own search to heal myself and radically improve my life has taken me far and wide, studying techniques ancient and contemporary, scientific and spiritual until it all came together within me. I desperately needed the answers that are in the methods I will share with you. I started searching for them before I was 10 years old. Even at such a young age, I was miserable and knew I didn't want to be miserable. I was driven to find answers. I remember staying up to 2 a.m. reading about a 2,500-year-old method for rebuilding one's health.

I've talked with dozens of doctors, nurse practitioners, nurses, and others in my search for help. By the time I got to the age when I needed to think about a career, I knew it made sense to get into health care, but it had to be outside of the mainstream medical model. Not because that model is bad but because I knew it didn't have the answers I was seeking.

I kept on my mission to figure out how to solve the problems I had by studying many forms of somatic therapies, yoga, martial arts, meditations, traditional forms of medicines, brain retraining techniques, and other methods. The answers I found came through combining the range of methods I learned and through training, research, experience with clients, and my own intuition.

It was important for me to go beyond simply being healthy. I wanted to know the upper end of what was possible. How could I find clarity? Feel energized? Have a positive sense of self? How could I make myself feel ecstatic?

The Nytality Method helped lead me to where I wanted to go.

I don't want this to sound as though I'm about to sell you a magic pill—these methods take real work and continuous effort to get results. You'll have to go deep within yourself and beyond yourself and to new levels of who and what you are. That isn't to say that what you will learn is difficult in the sense of rocket science or advanced mathematics, but focused, consistent attention over time presents its own challenges. It took me years to master this method myself, but it was worth the time and effort.

I've run a somatic therapy practice since 2002, helping people to approach their health holistically. I help people to work with their body, mind, and emotions, and have helped people with problems as small as sprained ankles and as complex as freeing themselves from past trauma that is still rooted in their body. I taught at a technical college for over five years, specializing in anatomy, physiology, psychology of success, and entrepreneurship. In addition to being the author of this series of books, I have been a guest on over 20 podcasts including "From Survivor to Thriver," "How to Not Get Sick and Die," and "Inner Voice" with Dr. Foojan Zeine.[3] I will be touring Europe to teach some of the methods in this book.

This book, in addition to my others, is designed to upgrade your hardware (brain, spine, and peripheral nerves) and software (your thoughts, habits, emotional tendencies) to give you a better functioning system, without the bugs that slow you down and make life harder than it needs to be.

THIS BOOK IS WRITTEN A BIT DIFFERENTLY

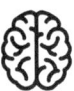

IN WRITING THIS BOOK, I organized the information in a way I believed would best deliver on my promise to give you specific methods to help your brain function better. I didn't realize how much my organizational style differs from that found in other books of this type until my writing coaches and editors pointed it out to me.

Where most authors would essentially set out all the big picture stuff up front and then go into more specifics and details in the back of the book, I have written *Un-F Your Brain and Be Happy* going back and forth between big general ideas and small specific ideas and practices. I did this because I want to encourage information transfer from the left hemisphere to the right hemisphere. The left side likes specifics and linear presentation of ideas and concepts, and the right side likes to work with big picture ideas and a less linear presentation to connect things in a more artistic way.

I want to help teach your brain not only to do left- and right-hemisphere thinking well but also to do them more consciously and to do them together in a more harmonious way. I have maintained that format throughout the book, so you will find that chapters go back and forth between specific actionable steps and practices for big picture ideas and concepts, and practices that are less direct and that work more with the "software" or basics of thinking and emotional habits.

I suggest working through the chapters as written to see if you can teach your brain to go back and forth: I believe that process is one of the secrets to thinking in a personally useful way, thinking differently, and shifting your emotions to a more positive state. However, if you prefer, feel free to go through the direct actionable chapters and put them all together and come back for the others later or do the big picture stuff first and come back to the direct actionable stuff later. Nothing in this book matters if you can't pull out the information and use it. So, by all means approach it in the way that works best for you. And have some fun while doing it. Fun makes things more sustainable long-term and if it's more sustainable, you'll get more out of it because you are still doing it.

ONE

WORKING WITH YOUR HARDWARE

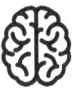

YOU CAN TAKE ANYTHING I present and make it work for you right here and right now. I've essentially created a library of methods to share; you are welcome to pick and choose what system you like and make it work for you.

Each of the 15 systems of the Nytality Method—this one included—has physical, mental, emotional, and energetic components, and each has methods to put the components together. Then, taken all together, the 15 systems come together as a program.

The system laid out in this book tackles working with and changing your mental and emotional states to live a healthier, happier life. In doing so, you will be able to expand your consciousness. It would be hard for me to accurately convey the radical mental, emotional, physical, and spiritual changes this system has provided for me.

The Nytality Method aims to be a user's manual for working on how you function and how to improve your inner state. It also aims to give you systematic methods to actively change your inner life through your own efforts.

So, what do I mean by inner state?

We experience different kinds of functioning based on our brain states, our neurochemistry, our hormones, our diets, our behaviors, our sleep, trance states, drugs, memories, and where we put our attention. In fact, I could easily make a case that everything you do, think, say, ingest, or have any control over is creating states within you.

Some of this is brain state-specific, which we will talk about in more depth later. But for now, the concept of "state" as I am using it here has to do with the quality of what is going on inside you mentally, emotionally, and consciously. Sometimes you are up, sometimes you feel down. Sometimes you feel sharp and clear, other times you feel slow and you struggle to put things together. Sometimes you experience your consciousness in a broad and expansive way, and at other times it seems narrow, limited, and dim.

The methods that I describe in this book are quite comprehensive and thorough. I will take you as far as possible in this book, and then we will take it further, if needed, in other books, courses, online classes, videos, and retreats.

It took me years to master this method myself, but it was worth the time and effort. I remember the time I finally achieved an ecstatic state. This happens when you reach the peak of what a human can become mentally, emotionally, physically, and energetically through an inner experience. It's something like a tree or plant flowering, something extraordinarily beautiful—but you experience it inside you.

An ecstatic state is created entirely inside you and can't be made by any external means. It's beyond emotions, mind, body, and life energy—rather it's a blossoming of all those things together within you. It's something a human can achieve through the right work within themselves. This state can heal you and make you whole again inside.

Nothing else in life comes close to this experience, at least not that I have tried or heard about. Drugs pretend to do it, and they certainly can give an experience that knocks you out of your normal experience of life, but they also limit your consciousness; you lose access to your ordinary consciousness while you use them. That is part of their appeal. They get you away from "yourself." But when you expand through consciousness methods, your ordinary consciousness stays with you.

I had read about ecstatic states before, but never dreamed they could be so powerful. The experience is mystical, transformative, and cosmically connecting. How do you put something that is so far beyond familiar dimensions into thoughts, words, symbols? Every part of you blossoms and opens up into a new fulfillment.

So, as I built my systems for the Nytality Method, I worked hard to construct them in such a way that everyday people could have that same experience. It requires conscious work and application to make it happen.

These changes have opened up my consciousness in ways beyond anything I could have possibly conceived. Now, I want to share them with you.

Questions to help apply and use the information in Chapter 1:

1. What do you see as the most obvious problem going on within you?
2. Is the problem within your mind, emotions, body, or maybe energy levels?
3. Can you see how working directly with your inner world could help your daily life get better?
4. What do you currently think or believe could get better for you?

TWO

SENSES MEDITATION

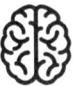

LET'S DIVE RIGHT INTO A method to get started.

To make use of the methods in this book you'll need to learn to get out of your logical, reasoning, judging, cutting-things-apart, intellectual mind. We've been trained to stay there almost all the time; people often can't shut their logical mind down even to be able to fall asleep.

We want to start by relearning how to use some of the other parts of us, like our consciousness. Consciousness is really more like a spectrum than an on/off switch, though many people experience it that way. Either it's turned all the way on and is running, or it's all the way off and asleep. But you learn to experience far more of the varying points on the spectrum through consciousness work. Doing so allows you to change how you experience yourself and life, it allows you to use more of your functions as a human being and it begins to help you have a different type of control over your life and experience.

These days we tend to experience our mind as a logical, reasoning machine with memory access, but the human mind is far grander and more capable. One aspect that we tend to miss developing is the non-logical, nonlinear part of our mind that doesn't connect through obvious 1-2-3-4-5 type relationships. For instance, its nonlinear connection might be something like 1–apple-game-want work to be fun-play-colorful-cartoon-story-call Bob about starting a manga creation studio.

It's not always easy to see the connections, and if you block that creative and connecting part of your mind, you'll miss the benefits. This part of you is usually trained out of you at school and at corporate jobs. It isn't easy for others to see or account for it and so it becomes a liability when people want to direct your action. It's also not very predictable and so the connections can sometimes feel like magic.

When you begin to drop your judging, intellectualizing, habitual, and largely automatic reflexes, you'll see that your mind, emotions, and consciousness can actually work for you in ways that you haven't learned to access well yet. For example, you might see that when you stop thinking about a problem for a while the answer shows up almost miraculously in your field of attention, as if another part of you entirely worked it out while you let your intellect rest and chill out.

But for most of us, at least in my observations, we have been trained to stay almost always in that judging, rationalizing, looking for problems, ego-protective sort of mental state. Of course, some of this is the natural animal part of us controlling the more human and complex part. (The ancient lizard in us stares at danger and drags our more human mental function into the endeavor.) You'll have to train this out of yourself. It's not about denying or pretending these aspects of you don't exist, you just bring them into line with your higher aspects.

Those powerful, older, ancient animal parts of you need to be part of the team but also need to be consciously in alignment with your higher functions. Nothing is suppressed because things that are suppressed will blow up. Rather they are part of the family and can be calmed because the high parts of you have them under control. The animal parts of you will be there when needed. For example, if you need to physically defend your life, they will be there.

Ultimately, we want to gain more conscious control of our analytical mind and our animal nature so that they work with us rather than controlling us and our inner consciousness.

So, let's start with an exercise to begin to calm those animal instincts and awaken other aspects of what we are in our consciousness and mind.

1. Find somewhere you can sit peacefully and safely without being interrupted. This step is important: how can you learn to calm your protective animal nature if you can't find somewhere to be safe for a few minutes?
2. Sit up straight. Reach the top of your head toward the sky.
3. Relax. Take a breath or two. Feel your body. Just experience it as there in your attention.
4. Put your attention on your eyes, not what you see but your actual physical eyes. Now close them.
5. Use your attention to work your way around your eyes, go front to back and relax them. Just let them let go. Take the stress and strain out of them. Let go. (Don't worry about what direction you move them—it's more important that it be relaxing. Do what works well for you.)
6. Now turn your attention to your ears. Feel them, and use your attention to work around them, top to bottom, side to side, just as you worked around your eyes.
7. Now move to your nose. Again, feel your way into it and up the passages a bit into your sinuses. Strip away the tension as your attention moves over them.
8. Move to your tongue. It's useful here to go back to front. Try to feel your tongue become heavy and then relax on the floor of your mouth.

9. Move down to both of your hands. Move your attention through your left hand, through the skin and nerves, going from wrist to fingers slowly and deliberately. Then move to your right hand and go through it thoroughly in the same way.
10. Now, if possible, endeavor to do eyes, ears, nose, tongue, and hands all together. You might need some practice on the individual parts before putting them all together.

None of this needs to be perfect, just play with it. Make it a beautiful pattern in your experience. Take it easy. It should be artistic rather than forced.

You may have noticed a pattern in these steps. We are looking to reduce attention on your five senses to open up your inner world to your consciousness. This is a key variable in accomplishing what we want to achieve with these methods. It's essential to get your attention and your consciousness inside you.

Most people have almost all their attention running through their senses into the outer world. To make these changes you need to be able to move your consciousness into your inner environment at will. Ultimately, that requires methods that rewire how you function, but gives amazing gifts that can't be accessed any other way. (We'll discuss some of these gifts in Chapter 6.) But for now, let me say that this will begin to change how you see yourself and experience the world in a very deep way. This allows you to change your mind, your emotions, your health, and your life.

[Note: To change your life, you have to change something in your life that you usually do. Changing the habits that make you "you" is essentially the access point to changing your life.]

In my opinion, the biggest change is how much agency you achieve over your own life experience. What I mean by that is you can begin, through your own inner efforts, to change how you feel, your emotions, your energy level, your mind, and your consciousness.

When I mention this to people, they often miss the importance of what will change for them. Imagine what would change if you could gain the ability to conduct your emotions. If you could feel elated inside without needing something to change outside of you. Imagine if you could generate more thoughts that you enjoyed thinking. Imagine if you could create 30% more usable energy for your life. Imagine if your consciousness became broader and clearer. Imagine if your sense of time changed to something more flexible so you could enjoy life more. Imagine if you could improve your memory and access to long-term memory.

How to start to apply the senses meditation:

(This is a recommended starting point but apply it any way that works for you.)

1. Run the senses meditation once a day for a week.
2. Keep a journal of how you *feel* before and after.

THREE

HOW THESE METHODS CAME ABOUT AND A HISTORY

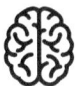

NOW THAT WE'VE HAD A taste of what we're getting ourselves into, let's move onto the big why of these methods, how they came about, and how they are built.

The big why? Desperation. Need. The need to find answers. And not just, "Well, it's the way it is," or "Life just sucks," or "It's just genetics, there's nothing I can do."

I was not going to give up until I found what I was looking for. And it was quite a journey inside and out to find the answers, to codify them in a way that works for me and figure out how to help others. From my perspective, I can't oversell these methods and the effect they have had on me and my life. Let me tell you about the journey I took to put these specific methods together and the Nytality Method in general. I'd like to share some context and perspective and how I reached for them.

In my first book, *Ah, Food, Why Do You Trouble Me So Much?* I spoke about the health problems I have but I'd like to expand on that here. Those issues are part of the puzzle I was trying to solve.

It wasn't until two years ago that I remember finally waking up without obvious pain. Even as a kid I was in pain. Headaches, joint pain, tooth pain, tissue pain, stomach pain, intestinal pain, temperature control issues, incredible mind fog (which was itself painful), ringing ears, massive unrelenting fatigue and exhaustion, bloody noses, night terrors, depression, anxiety, and a few other problems I'll keep to myself. A great deal of this suffering had to do with some infections I had picked up. And some had to do with trauma I experienced, which I will talk about later. Now, I work with clients who complain of many of the same things.

Most of the well-meaning doctors I spoke with had no answer for me, the same with the nurse practitioners. By the time I was 12, I knew I would have to figure out these health problems largely on my own. So, I started reading about any kind of health methods I could find. I didn't care where the information came from, how old or new, how difficult or different from my preconceived notions. Over time, I was willing to look at everything. Often, I'd be up all night reading things. I'd be in unusual sections of libraries and bookstores. Looking back, I can see that for me the pain and suffering acted as a whip to prod me along.

I never completely gave up on looking for help from medical practitioners, and eventually I found some great help there too. The combination of my own methods and those of the medical and health practitioners I saw got me to a good place with my health.

The particular problems I had were hard to find in books, hard to diagnose, and hard to kill off. Progress in diagnoses and cures has improved over the years but there is still misunderstanding and misinformation. I was bitten by a tick when I was four or five. The first bite gave me a few different infections, rather unusual ones that caused a lot of problems for me over the years. Because of these initial infections, my immune system was weakened. That allowed for a whole host of other infections to gain access to my system. Over the years, I think I have been through treatment for around 14 infections, including Lyme, Bartonella, Rickettsia, a number of gut parasites, surgical infections, and West Nile, to name a few.

If you were to look at the reported symptoms of these infections, you'd see that they show up in an extraordinary number of different ways. This is in large part why they are so hard to diagnose. These infections, as I was told by several doctors, often come together from the same bite and then leave you susceptible to more. Testing for things like Lyme is tricky. There are many kinds, and they don't always show up on standard blood tests. So, you can see how they are hard to find and diagnose. Many people don't show the obvious symptoms, like the bullseye rash of Borrelia, the spots of a certain kind of Rickettsia, or the stretch-mark looking signs of Bartonella. I had two of the three, but when I was a kid, I didn't know that. I remember thinking, why do I have stretch marks so young? But I didn't know then that I was sick.

In the early stages, the treatment for these diseases is pretty simple. But it gets trickier if you wait, like I did.

Perhaps you can see why I was desperately trying to find answers as I grew older. Healing, in a deep way, is a rather large process that can involve way more than you might think. This led me to study a wide range of subjects from medical journals to yoga to meditation to visceral manipulation to social dynamics to learned childhood behaviors and trauma.

If the solution to your health problems isn't obvious, you might have to cast a wider net to learn how to boost the natural healing processes of your mind, emotions, body, energy, and spirit. But many answers lie in those areas.

We've been conditioned by the brilliance of modern medicine to think that everything is easily fixable with a pill or surgery. And many things are. But there are also many health problems that require you to work more broadly with yourself: your mind, your body, your emotions, your will, and your attention.

Let me see if I can give you a simple, easy-to-follow example of what I mean.

Every day that I go into the clinic where I work, I know I will see people with neck pain. People expect to come in and have me help fix the pain in their neck with manual methods. And of course, I will do that. But many people I work with don't realize just how much they are working against themselves because of the way they use their mind and emotions. So many of them are in such a hurry to feel better, they don't address the root cause of their problem. People who are stressed, in a hurry, trying to please others, who expect "no pain no gain," people who can't stop imagining bad things in the future, people who dwell on bad things in the past, and people who are anxious—are stiff. Their muscles are shortened in the soft tissues, putting extra pressure on their circulatory system to push through the tension, inhibiting the flow of lymph fluid. Their heartbeat often races, and they exhibit other physical signs of what is going on inside.

These things pull on the neck and head causing tension, which causes eventual pain and weakness (because the muscles are worn down from the constant battle to hold up your head up against stress and tension and gravity), potential heart strain, jaw pain, and so on.

You end up using your autonomic nervous system and staying most of the time in the sympathetic branch of the system rather than parasympathetic branch which would allow you to do things like rest, digest, rebuild, and repair your system. After years of that, you want the therapist to fix the problem with two hours of work over two weeks.

I often have 25 total minutes with people on the table. I'll see someone fly into the parking lot 45 seconds before the appointment and run into the building literally huffing and puffing when they get on the table, stiff as a board, mind racing and all of that. It'll take me, even with really cool techniques to help them switch to that relaxed state, probably three to five minutes just to settle them down.

Now, I'm not making fun of anyone. Most of us have been trained to live like this. Almost everyone you see is this way. It's rare to see someone who can stay fluid in the flow of their life so that their nervous system can switch back and forth at will from rest and rebuild to on and dealing with things that need super focus or actually involve some sort of danger. But you can learn to live in this fluid state and access varying degrees of flow state. It's not that you need to be a passive and non-engaged person. It's that you want to have the right conditions for the right timing to have the best life possible.

Learning to live that kind of life requires an overall holistic view of life: how you treat yourself, how you conduct your time (or how it uses you), how you use your mind (or how it uses you), how you conduct your emotions (or how they control you), and most importantly, how you use your attention (or how your attention is used by your environment and everyone else).

Going back to my description of people frantically running into the clinic, what do you think happens when people live that way for a long time? What happens to their health, their mental health, their emotional health, their epigenetics (factors that turn genetic patterns off and on), and their life experience? Maybe you can understand why I began to look everywhere and at everything to try to solve my health problems. Complex, chronic, and complicated problems often require solutions beyond a pill or surgery (although they might also require those as part of the picture). I was willing to look everywhere.

As my search evolved, I realized my physical health problems weren't the only problems I needed to solve. I needed to work though some significant childhood trauma that complicated my life with nightmares, hypervigilance, and more.

The methods I've outlined in this book are the single best set of tools I have found. They have radically changed what my inner experience has been in relation to traumatic events. And my belief is they can and will do the same for many of you too. Whether you have been through some truly f'ed up stuff or you have had any exposure to life with trauma, disconnect, and discomfort, these methods might be exactly what you are looking for to improve your inner and outer life.

But let's talk a bit about what happened…

Questions to help you move forward from here:

(One thing to recognize is that your feelings and beliefs really do matter.)

1. Do you feel right now that you want a change in you and in your life enough to take some kind of action? Can you see yourself doing it regularly?

2. Do you believe that you can actually change yourself or your life through your own efforts? If not, why not? Did someone else give you the idea that life can't be changed? Or did someone else convince you that you specifically can't change?

FOUR

TRAUMA DIRECTLY AFFECTS YOUR BRAIN AND CENTRAL NERVOUS SYSTEM

ONE OF THE MAJOR IMPULSES for this work comes from some intense and traumatic things that happened when I was a child, before I turned 12.

Heavy-duty trauma—particularly inflicted by someone purposely messing with your mind and emotions as well as your body—has a lasting impact. People often dismiss how bad mental and emotional violence is. Somehow, we have it confused. Society often thinks physical violence is the only violence, but in my opinion, the emotional and mental violence is harder to find and harder to heal.

Don't worry, I'm not going to go anywhere too graphic. I just want to talk about trauma and its effects on someone when under particularly intense pressure, especially when that pressure is consciously and deliberately applied. It can really change how you function now and forever.

I mentioned this history briefly in my second book, *Ah, Brain, Why Do You Trouble Me So Much?* but I'll add a little bit here. I unfortunately knew and was the prey of a child molester, who also happened to be a serial killer. His equally manipulative and sadistic daughter was involved, too.

They were genius manipulators who were 20 chess moves ahead of everyone else. Because of the threats to my family, I kept silent — I didn't tell a soul until decades later when I finally opened up to my therapist. Part of the reason I never told anyone is because the terror I felt from watching those people when I was young grew and matured into something out of a horror movie. You know those horror movies where, if you say the name of the evil, the evil shows up? That's how it felt—and still feels—in my mind. Even though neither of those people is alive today, I still feel that fear. Even typing this, I feel my body squirm.

But I know for sure that those two monsters are no longer alive and the threat no longer exists, so now I can share more of the lessons that time in my life gave me. During that time, I was desperate to survive. And I did—with my mind and heart intact. This is a big part of why the methods in this book now exist and why I know they work even under very trying circumstances.

In its entirety, the Nytality Method is, in a sense, a method to break free—from terrible things, yes, but also from smaller, everyday things. It's a beautiful answer to the question, how does one heal and move forward from such trauma? It's worked amazingly for me, and I hope it will for you, too. This is a good time to mention that qualified therapy can be invaluable for you if you are struggling with trauma or anything difficult. You don't have to go it alone. There are wonderful people trained and passionate to help you.

It's the choices that you make—most importantly the choices you make inside you—that determine what your life will be like. What thoughts do you harbor, what emotions do you dwell on, what actions do you take or not take? Are you able to break the habits you have created to wake up the real you?

I'm not saying it's easy—it takes more of you than anything else I can imagine. But nothing is more valuable. It takes every part of you coming together and moving in the same general direction. It takes your mind, your emotions, your feelings, your body, your dark or shadow side, your attention, and your consciousness. You bring all these aspects of yourself together and then work on them consciously and repeatedly.

I joke a bit about what it feels like to turn your inner "computer" off and on again but that is very much what it feels like to me. It helps to shut down programs that have been running open in the background that you aren't entirely aware of but that are still having an effect on you. I also think it creates a pause for you to do a system check on the nervous system because everything gets quiet enough for that part of you to work behind the scenes. In this case, I actually mean the hardware within your central and peripheral nervous systems as well as the software: the thoughts, emotions, and belief systems you are running.

Life itself can be so intense that the average person can never get the chance for a real reset to happen. Unfortunately, if you've been through some significant trauma—whatever that means for you—you are almost certainly stuck with systems and programs running that will never turn off without a specific method to accomplish this. The Nytality Activating Methods as a whole do this brilliantly.

It's fair to say these methods saved me and my experience of life from being stuck in the past, stuck in fear, stuck in anxiety, stuck in hypervigilance, and just plain stuck in life.

These methods give you some power back over yourself. You get to reclaim more of who and what you are.

For me, it's a personal flex and middle finger back to those who purposely tried to damage me, my mind, my heart, and my life.

I set myself free through my own efforts.

I'm not saying I don't still have mental and emotional scars but I can say I have radically healed myself and that has wonderful meaning for me and tells me who I really am.

It's my sincere wish that these methods will do that for you too.

FIVE

DEBUGGING YOUR MENTAL SOFTWARE

"EVERYONE KNOWS YOU HAVE TO have a whole potato with every meal, Todd."

This matter-of-fact assertion is made by my suffering client, who's lying face down on the physical therapy table.

"Wait a minute," I said, "everyone knows what?"

"Everyone knows that a healthy person eats a whole potato with every meal."

I wondered if, somehow, she could *feel* the bewildered look on my face. Because the ferocity with which she had made her pronouncement stunned me as if someone had caught me with a surprise left hook.

"My grandmother taught me right," she went on. "Don't try to convince me that I need to change my diet or how I eat!"

"Yes, but you can barely walk anymore," I said as gently as possible. "And your blood pressure is dangerously high."

"Look, I know you are going to say that because I am 200 pounds overweight that's part of the reason my knees and hips can barely hold me up. Just like my doctor said. But this has nothing to do with weight. Do your job and fix my knees. And my blood pressure."

She said this with an air of final authority. The subject was closed as far as she was concerned.

At this point, I was less concerned about her knees than I was about her brain. Carefully, I tried to break down this buggy notion she'd been holding on to for probably fifty years or more.

"I'll do my best," I said, "but please consider rethinking what your grandma told you. She can be both the greatest woman you've ever met and also wrong with some of the advice she gave. Her advice might have been appropriate for farmers working 12- to 16-hour days 365 days a year. But it might not be quite right today."

Have you noticed how many people seem to be really struggling with daily life? Like life itself is a burden. That life is something to be suffered through, with a few breaks of pleasure here and there until it ends.

Another way to express my meaning here is how many people do you know personally who are having a wonderful time in their daily life? (By the way, don't confuse people you know personally with people cleaning up and sanitizing their daily life for social media and appearances edited to look like they are doing well.)

Outside of when you were actually a kid, do you have friends, family, or coworkers who are having the kind of wonderful time that we often associate with the innocence of childhood?

If you are anything like almost everyone I've ever talked to, your mind will be screaming at me things like:

"Kids don't have to work!"

"It's only fools who don't see how painful life is!"

"If you knew my history, you'd understand how crazy your head-in-the-clouds, flighty ass sounds."

"Life is meant to be suffered, until you die and get your reward after all the suffering, pain and drama."

"There are people suffering all over the world, if I'm happy it's selfish and somehow belittling the people in other places."

"No pain, no gain."

"Life sucks and then you die."

"If I were king, I would fix it all and make it all right."

"No one loves me."

"Everyone is taking advantage of me."

"No one respects me."

"Life isn't fair."

"Only the rich are happy."

"Old age is the worst!"

"When you get to my age, you'll see."

"Who do you think you are to be happy?"

Essentially, it's all happening outside of me and is someone else's fault.

But why?

Are the people you know suffering because they are starving? Are they chained to a wall in the hell that is slavery? Are they being actively, physically tortured by a razor-wielding psychopath? Are they rotting from the inside out from some unknown disease/s?

Please make no mistake, some people are in those situations, and I don't wish any of them on you or me. I do know what it's like to be chained to a wall in a basement and in a school. I do know what it's like to be rotting from the inside out from some weird diseases. I know what it's like to have someone play with my emotions and mind to cause me pain and suffering. I'm not making light of people in those situations. Hell resides closely within them.

However, even then you have choices. Even then you have a beautiful and powerful mind. Especially then your emotions can be your best friend, or they can be your nightmare.

The suffering is inside you.

Pain is a different story, although it's still something you can work with. I'm essentially making a distinction between physical pain and mental and emotional suffering like many before me. Epictetus does an interesting job of discussing this topic as does Viktor Frankl in *Man's Search for Meaning*.

On the flip side though, this also means that happiness, bliss, ecstasy, and satisfaction are within you too. I'm not trying to say that you shouldn't want a better life. In fact, I think you should work passionately toward what you would define as a better life. But I do want to suggest that maybe you shouldn't make your outer life 95% of your happiness, bliss, ecstasy, and satisfaction. I think you should flip the ratio.

I'm also not trying to suggest that you give up working on your outer world or dream life. Interestingly, I think it works the opposite from what you probably believe. Your outer life will improve when you definitively change your inner life to something better.

I question deeply the belief that your outer world is 100% separate from your inner subjective life. I actually see a correlation and even a direct connection. I believe, and it definitely is my experience, that what is going on inside you radiates into your outer environment. And so, working on your inner world changes your outer world over time too.

The problem for most is that they let their outer life rule their inner life. That means they let the influences of the outer world set what is going on within them, and the power of their mind, emotions, energy, and focus makes that influence set up their outer world. It becomes a loop that leads them to having the same life all the time. The same problems keep coming around and often growing as they pick up momentum.

So, breaking this cycle is the crux of changing your life and life experience. It's extraordinarily important that you begin to take control of your inner life through your own consciousness and efforts. Otherwise, the same cycles will go on and on and on.

You have to change something to get something new.

Okay, so if the reason for your suffering is not that you're starving or in incredible physical pain, what is causing the suffering? Couldn't you then say it's a product of what's going on within your mind, emotions, energy, health, and the way you run yourself?

This point tends to upset people, because it implies a lot of things that people don't want to hear. I understand that, and I'm not making fun of you or saying that bad things haven't happened to you. I'm actually trying to give you a message of hope, because it means things can change through your efforts.

At this point shame, blame, and guilt have to be addressed. These emotions will keep you from being able to clearly see what's going on and where cause and effect lies and to find the path to where you want to go. These emotions at this point will turn off your logical and reasoning mind. They will also distort your memory and how you remember things happening. Enormous manipulation and control are wielded over people through these emotions.

Please keep in mind, however, that you do need a barometer for wrongdoing. It takes a while to figure out through your own inner compass where you stand in relationship to the question of wrongdoing. Everyone needs to be able to fit within their society. They need to understand laws, morals, and ethics, but a great deal of pressure that's been applied to you has been in the name of control over you, your actions, your mind, and your emotions—not to create a functioning society, but to give someone power over you.

I'm not trying to give you permission to break laws, harm people, or create general anarchy. What I am trying to point out is that people have laid hundreds of emotional bombs within you through shame, guilt, and blame, and it will take real effort to get to the point where you can function without these unconscious emotions limiting you and your life.

Every person I have known who has changed their life for the better through their own efforts seems to work on the principle that everything in their life is a result of those efforts. They take responsibility. Now, if you apply the emotions of shame, blame, and guilt, the emotions will take over your mind. Perhaps you will run to the extreme and call me a victim blamer and throw this book away and tell everyone I'm evil or bad.

The universe is big and complex and there are many variables within the equation of how things happen, to whom they happen, when they happen, and so on. But what this idea of taking responsibility for your life does is empower you. Because now you can work as if there is some cause and effect in the universe. Without any cause and effect, you are lost. Lost in a universe that is just spinning with no rhyme, reason, mathematics, or logic.

An interesting thing seems to happen as I watch people go to the "life is completely random, or God hates me" place. Depression takes over, energy disappears, overall health declines, people begin to attack themselves—physically, mentally, and emotionally. Much of how you function is created by neurotransmitters in response to your ability to accomplish, to find meaningful relationships, and to work to make your life better and see some progress in that direction.

If you believe there's no cause and effect and that you can do nothing, be nothing, or change nothing to make you or your life better, how can you possibly regulate your emotions? How can you regulate the energy that you experience in your daily life? How can you direct your mind that believes nothing matters and that is lost in confusion and an inability to connect anything in life?

With all that going on inside, you'll never be able to make your life better. And so, starting with taking responsibility to take things where they are now and move them forward gives you ground to stand on. It does not absolve evil, manipulative, violent, lawbreaking, molesting, murdering, kidnapping people who might have done things, even to you. *They* did those things, not you. You don't ever take responsibility for what other people did because you can't control them.

Evil people are gonna evil.

So, you take responsibility for doing everything you can to keep yourself safe, protected, emotionally healthy, mentally healthy, physically healthy, and you especially use your attention to the best of your ability to put yourself in positions to be safe and successful.

Be wise. Be wise about what you do, what you think, what you say, where you are, why you are there, how you conduct your emotions, and how your ego drives you.

If you do these things, you'll stay clear of all kinds of evil people evil-ing. You might still get caught in something—in that case, do the very best you can with what you have available. Create boundaries. Stand up for yourself when necessary. Get help if you can.

And remember this because this saved my life on numerous occasions: You are more powerful than you know. You have no idea what you can do or create or your ability to defend yourself until you unleash yourself.

You need to know when to unleash yourself and how to unleash. These times are very rare; when your ego is bruised is not the time. When your life and freedom are on the line, that's when you unleash the beast within you—wisely.

Now let's address the elephant in the room. What do you do if you're chained to a wall and can't get out literally or figuratively? What do you do if your body, mind, and emotions are rotting around you?

I have been in both situations in the case of health problems for decades. What you have at that moment is your attention and your consciousness. In fact, when you are in that situation is when you are really introduced to your consciousness and your attention.

The power that is there is beyond anything you can imagine. And what you have control over at that moment is to work the best you can with your mind, emotions, energies, and body. You still have a choice, you still have power, you can still do something even if at that moment you can't control what's going on with your body.

I pray none of you find yourself in those experiences.

It's partly because of these moments that I deeply question the idea that our inner subjective life is absolutely separate from our outer objective life. Because when that was all I had, I could still impact my outer life through activity in my inner world. Things changed because of what I did inside.

Your inner world matters. Both the inside and outside of you always matter.

That is just the beginning of why you should work on these methods. They grow within you into something beyond what you can now believe possible.

They introduce you to more of yourself. They help you connect with the greatest parts of yourself. And this connection changes everything in your experience. This is part of the reason that lots of old methods were focused on ego: it keeps you from getting in contact with the greatest part of you and recognizing the power and beauty of that realization.

The Nytality Method is aimed at making your connection with the greatest parts of yourself come to fruition. This connection will heal, rebuild, uplift, and remake your life experience. The specific techniques in this book begin a deep process for changing how your mind works, how your emotions function, how you experience yourself and your consciousness. The techniques provide a map and method to begin to reprogram your mind, nervous system, brain states, and to help break you free from the way your nervous system and mind have been functioning. The method is a reset button when you are stuck in sympathetic mode, when you can't make a change inside on your own.

| Questions to help you debug:

1. Can you see the value in debugging your mental and emotional software?
2. What do you think would be the overall change you might experience by going through old ideas that you haven't challenged thoroughly?
3. Every day try to find one old idea that you are clinging to that might be holding you back now. Are you able to prove it false? Challenge it.

SIX

THE POWER BREATH

NEVER MIND

ONE DAY I RECEIVED AN unexpected message from one of my longest-running clients. We'll call her Linda (not her real name). I say it was unexpected because Linda had moved hours away and I hadn't seen her in a long time.

She told me she had a number of issues she needed my help with. Since I had last seen her, she said, she had been through a range of difficult experiences, including the loss of multiple family members. She was reaching out to me, she said, because of how much I'd helped her in the past.

On the day of her appointment, she drove hours to see me, and when she walked in, I could tell she was as happy to see me as I was to see her. Sitting in my office, she asked if I could help her with the anxiety and anger she felt about what had happened in her life.

There are a range of techniques within acupressure, craniosacral therapy, and visceral manipulation that can be quite helpful for a person in Linda's situation. But they are somewhat limited because once the techniques have been applied and the session is over, the person can continue generating anxiety and anger depending on where they put their attention and what they think about.

I like to think I'm good at what I do, but I know I will never be able to get ahead of someone with their brain and nervous system essentially stuck in worry and anger mode. Fortunately, the methods in my system do offer tools for resetting the nervous system and allowing people to rework the programs running in their mind, emotions, and body.

I told Linda about the tools, how they work, and how much they could help her get out of her current mode. She was excited and receptive.

"Go ahead and do them to me!" she said.

Carefully, I explained to her, again, that these were methods I could teach her, but she would have to put them into practice. Her body visibly stiffened at hearing she would have to apply the methods herself.

"Oh, okay," Linda said, visibly irritated with me, "then never mind."

I had a good solution for her problem—something she could do in three to five minutes a day—that could have made a positive, long-term difference in her life. But that solution wasn't what she anticipated. It required an effort from her.

Unfortunately, this is a common occurrence in my world. Most people are looking for someone to hand the solution to them or provide it for them. They reject things that could help their problem simply because it requires some sort of change or action on their part, especially if that change or action is outside their habits, automatic thoughts, and usual range of emotions or behaviors.

Taking a little initiative and doing the work on your own is the only way to solve many problems. My methods wouldn't be here if I hadn't had to find my own way to the solutions I needed. My methods only work if you learn them and do them, and there is only a little value in knowing *how* to do them—the real solution is in the *doing*.

When you are feeling depleted or anxious, the following breathing exercise is a great help. It is a simple exercise that we want to do for several reasons, which I list at the end of the exercise. To start, we want to super-oxygenate the system. I first saw a version of this kind of breathing in a martial arts video when I was a kid. Later, I saw similar exercises in martial arts schools, and I believe it is close to one of the techniques of Wim Hof [4] (although I haven't studied with him to see for myself). Often, you'll find that versions of valuable practices show up all over the world as practitioners find different ways to access that value for themselves.

The power breath

1. Take a moment to relax, get yourself in the moment, and then get into your body. Actually feel your body with your attention and consciousness.
2. Take in a deep, quick breath—like you are sucking in extra oxygen.
3. Pull that air toward your lungs and then up toward your brain. (At first your abdomen expands during the in breath, then you gently push your abdomen in and your breath up. Feel your breath go toward your brain.) This is a feeling exercise as much as a breathing exercise. You are encouraging a change in your system although you aren't actually pushing oxygen into your brain.
4. Don't push out as much air as you take in; just a simple exhalation.
5. Repeat 30 times.
6. On the last repeat, hold the breath gently, in and up as if the air is fueling your brain directly. [7]) Let it out when it feels like you are just about

to really need a breath. Don't force the hold but let it last for a while.

This method is really powerful for making a change throughout your system and was essential to me in the recovery of my health and energy levels. You can do it three times in a row up to three times a day. But don't force it. Breathing exercises are powerful in ways that influence your nervous system as well as body chemistry. Don't force them. Go slow, take your time. If the exercise feels bad or painful, stop immediately. Trust your body and intuition.

Specific results I recognize from this exercise:

1. Memory retrieval
2. More useful daily energy
3. Better sleep
4. Improved ability to wake up
5. Quieting of the mind/improved clarity in thought, reasoning, and finding connections.
6. Reduction and (for long periods of time) complete removal of anxiety
7. Alleviation of depression
8. Recreated states of joy, bliss, and ecstasy (I am making a distinction here that these are not a single emotional state but rather have differences in how good they feel as well as differences in energy and physical experience.)
9. Alleviation of headaches
10. Reduction in neck and shoulder pain
11. Significant increase in occurrence, depth, and duration of synchronicities
12. Improved ability (in time, capacity, and depth) to perform work
13. Improved sense of and appreciation of self
14. Significant reduction in concern about what others think of me and my life

I think that most of the results stated above are available to anyone. I attribute many of the improvements I saw in my problems with infections to the healing effects of this method, which helped my brain, nervous system, neurotransmitters, and hormones. My vision improved as did all my other senses. There were significant improvements.

How to practice the power breath:

Try practicing this when you wake up in the morning, even before you leave your bed. See if it adds a little spring to your step. Also try it in the afternoon when you feel like you are starting to move a little slower.

SEVEN

A DESPERATE NEED

DO YOU EVER GET THE feeling that if you could improve what is going on inside of you that everything in your life would improve?

Is anyone else desperate to improve their life?

I used to think everyone felt this way, but I realized after talking to people and watching how they function that many people aren't actually thinking or acting in this way at all. Let me be clear: I think—deep down—everyone wants a better life but surprisingly few endeavor to make it happen. Many don't believe it's possible. Many think the only way to improve their life and feel better in the hierarchical part of their brain is to control and "alpha" others. Some think life is against them, God hates them, or fate has wrecked them. Essentially, it seems to me that many people feel like they are powerless and have no agency in their life or even in themselves.

That has never made any sense to me. Not even for a second did I ever believe that line of thinking. So, for me, I just had to figure out how to do it. Then, once I saw it and understood it, I could codify and execute it. This idea pursued me and drove me to great lengths and efforts to figure it out and make it happen for my own inner life and daily life.

I remember talking to an old friend of mine. I would say, of all the friends I've ever had, she has the most "life is randomly happening" attitude, resigned to a complete lack of personal agency. She said, "I don't know how you do these things I've seen you do. It's like magic"—with clear disbelief and cognitive dissonance in her face, tone, and words. To her, it's unbelievable that someone could improve their life, make things happen, and follow a direction until achievement is reached in an obvious way. Her belief is that everything just happens without anyone doing anything. Life is a cosmic mistake with no purpose, meaning, laws, or predictability. She is even on the fence as to whether or not humans have any free will.

And she suffers.

She obviously suffers as she can't regulate her emotions, she can't see her efforts amounting to anything, she can't get herself to do the things that would change her life for the better. She lives out the beliefs she holds, and they make her life more painful for her.

I hope no one sees this as an attack—this friend is someone I care for deeply. It hurts my heart to see her live out that belief system. It may seem like I am talking about something that is "pie-in-the sky thinking" but I see taking charge of your life as absolutely essential in determining the kind of life you have and the way you experience it. I actually see this as the most practical thing you can do.

You will live out the programming in your heart and mind, like a program run in a supercomputer. Even if it's the fastest, most powerful, and most connected computer ever created, a self-defeating program will create a problem. And the faster the computer, the faster the program will self-destruct. Many smart people blow up their lives quickly because their minds are applying the program faster and more efficiently than a person who is not as smart could do it. It can be a curse to have a fast mind and a poorly designed program running in it.

So far as I can tell, if you want to improve your life, it's essential to work through your programming, either through your own efforts or with a qualified counselor. Most of this programming was installed in you when you were young. That means you didn't have the faculties to reject it through critical thinking and the wisdom of experience.

I address that issue at length in *Ah, Brain, Why Do You Trouble Me So Much?* so I won't dwell on it here, but one of the important aspects of the work addressed in *this* book is its ability to get under the programming. As your mind slows down and even becomes silent, the programming stops, and you have the ability to see what the programs are. The emotionality behind them stops and things become clear. Then you can rebuild the programming in a new way. This is one of the greatest benefits the work in this book has offered me and can also offer you. It's a truly extraordinary experience to feel your mind quiet and to discover how much turbulence it is constantly creating within your consciousness. We're not there yet, but the methods in this book can lead you closer if not all the way there. I hope a few of you will follow them that far. It's truly beautiful.

But most people are far more interested in changing their life right here and now and getting control of their inner world—their mind, emotions, energies, and body—is the most fundamental place to start. These are the mechanisms through which you experience your life. They create how your attention and consciousness allow you to experience life. So, if they are out of control and attacking you, then no matter what you change in your life you will continue to suffer because the suffering is being manufactured inside. You could win the lottery and be miserable. You could have the best romantic partner and love and be incredibly depressed. You could be adored the world over and wish to end yourself.

You have to change what's going on within you. It's what determines what is going on within your consciousness. This is essential.

The methods in this book will help you see what's going on inside by calming everything down so you can look at what is actually happening and then rewire and rewrite yourself. They provide a good start for changing yourself and, over time, that will radiate into every aspect of your life.

Questions to ask yourself:

1. Do you believe taking some responsibility for how you feel and how you function inside could make your life better?
2. Do you like to give away responsibility for what is going on within you to others?
3. Does this help you guilt, shame, and infuriate others into changing their behavior?
4. Can you see that you might be hurting yourself to try to control other people's behavior?

EIGHT

CASCADE MEDITATION

ALL RIGHT, ONTO THE NEXT step in the Vital Brain Method:

The Cascade Meditation

1. Find some time and somewhere quiet to practice.
2. Sit up straight, roll your hips slightly forward, reach the top of your head toward the sky and feel it lightly held up at the crown of your head.
3. Take a few minutes to let everything relax and let your breathing become slow and deep. Don't force any of this.
4. Direct your attention toward the crown of your head, the very top or where the soft spot was when you were a baby. Gently hold that attention for 30 seconds to a minute.
5. Draw your attention down the center of your forehead to the space between your eyebrows. Draw a line there with your attention—feeling it in your body—as the line goes from point to point in a relaxed, slow, and deliberate way.
6. Draw your attention from the point between your eyebrows straight

back toward the back of your head and your pituitary gland.

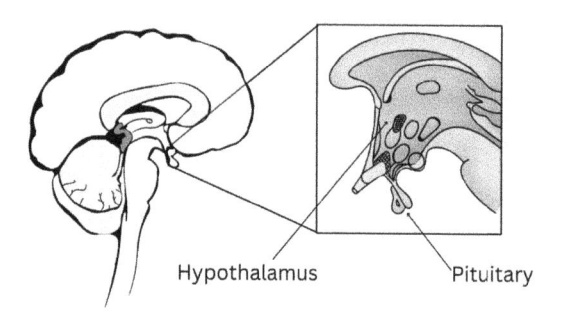

Hypothalamus   *Pituitary*

Pituitary & hypothalamus

7. Run your attention through the gland to activate and relax it. Activation here means to wake it up through your attention—you don't need anatomical understanding of the gland to do this work. Your nervous system already knows where the gland is and how to reach it. You just need to reconnect to what is already known subconsciously. Intellectualizing and getting lost in your memory are the opposite of what we want to accomplish here. We actually want to give the intellect a break, to slow down, and we want to free ourselves from the demands of memory.

8. Now that we have activated the pituitary gland, we will move further toward the back of the head to reach the pineal gland.[5]

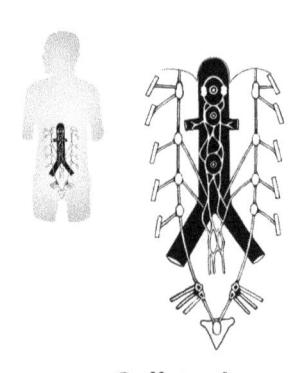

Celiac plexus

9. Activate the pineal gland by running your attention through it. These activations may or may not actually produce a physical sensation. Don't worry about either; all you want at this point is to create the sense of the connections in yourself.
10. Draw your attention forward again to the space between your eyes and then lead it down over your nose, mouth, and chin to reach the front of your neck. Here we find the thyroid gland roughly at the center.
11. Run your attention through the thyroid until you feel satisfied that you did it thoroughly. Again, don't force anything. There are no grades, no one is watching—this is your gig. Make it feel good and work for you. This won't work if you strain.
12. Draw your attention from the center of your throat down to where your collar bones meet, and you'll find the top of the sternum and the thymus gland.

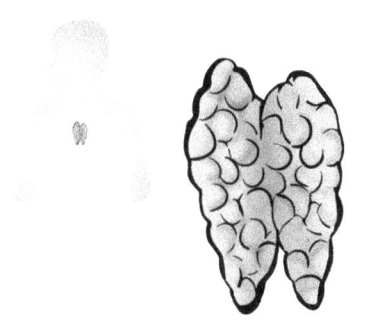

Thymus

13. Lead your attention through your thymus to wake up and activate this gland. Your mind and attention are way more powerful than you might think when you direct them onto different aspects of your body. This will have some interesting effects on you, your emotions, your mind, and ultimately your consciousness. Most people never experience this because they've always directed most of their attention to the outside world. Trying to control that, they have missed the power of working

inside themselves.

14. After working with the thymus in a satisfying way, take your attention further down your torso to the lower side of your sternum where there is no bone. Now, lead your attention back toward your spine until you almost reach it. Here you will find the celiac plexus.

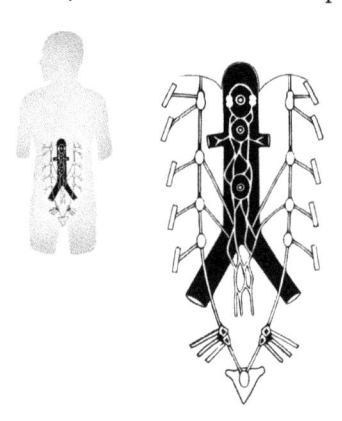

Celiac plexus

15. Work your mind and attention through the celiac plexus until you have satisfyingly created the activation you are looking for or at least until you feel comfortable to move on. Adequate is good enough, perfectionism will block what you are trying to create here.

16. Draw your attention down from the celiac plexus straight toward your hips until you reach your kidneys, on top of which you will find your adrenal glands.

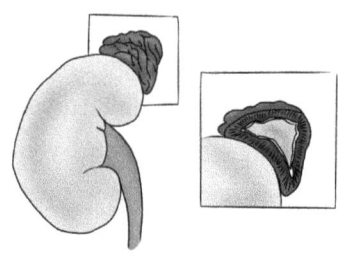

Adrenal gland

17. Bisect your attention toward both adrenal glands at the same time and again run your attention through the glands until you feel satisfied, like you've gotten something done. Nice and easy—nothing serious is going on here—you're just getting something useful to happen inside.
18. Move your attention further down into your pelvis until you reach your testes or ovaries. If you have had your ovaries removed, just do this in your imagination.

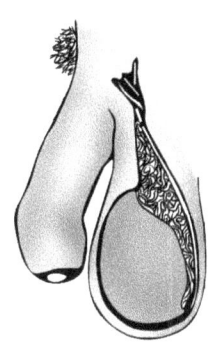

Testes

19. With as much ease and relaxation as possible, run your attention through your ovaries or testicles until you feel like you're done. No strain, no seriousness, no pain, no grades, no perfectionism, no performing—just play with the process.
20. Now sit and relax; try not to jump up and rush off unless you absolutely have to. It's good to take a few minutes to let your nervous system absorb and reflect the changes you've just made so they can become more permanent in your experience.

People often are in a constant state of rush and hurry; they don't know how to shut it all down and access the other parts of themselves. This is a point that can be hard to get across to people because we have been taught a way of being—a combination of how we use our body, mind, emotions, and time. It is so embedded for most people that it seems like how life is. This meditation will help you learn to shut all of that down and begin again from a different place. You don't need to be in a hurry all the time, and when you are you are cutting yourself off from different aspects of your mind, emotions, and body. If you can learn to quiet everything down, these aspects will come alive for you. They will add a beautiful and powerful flavor to your life.

How to work with the Cascade Meditation:

Practice this method daily and keep a journal to see how you feel before and after. Write it down so you can see what changes you might be experiencing. This might take a little while. Seek a change in how you feel, one that leads to a general relaxation and sense of calm.

NINE

MEDITATIVE STATES

IN LARGE PART, THE METHODS in this book could be considered a form of meditation or gaining control over your brain states. The term meditation can be tricky because it conjures up a lot of preconceived notions ranging everywhere from relaxation techniques, holding postures, religion, spirituality, universal absorption, and even hocus-pocus. But it is all about the experience. That is where, and only where, the magic of it lies. Naming it, or even understanding it intellectually, won't make any changes for you.

But I do want to broach the subject a bit here. To do these exercises you learn to first sit up straight with your eyes closed to work inside yourself. The process can definitely give you an altered state of awareness and change your emotional states. I believe this has a large effect on your brainwaves moving from high Beta to low Beta to Alpha and into the ranges of Delta, Theta, and Gamma. I don't know, of course, because I have been focused on making the methods work for me in my life right now and haven't yet started seeking scientific data to support it through brain scans. Someday I do hope to move in that direction, though.

Ultimately, learning how to achieve these states and experience them became a deep search for me. I wanted to find a way to codify and organize them and then build my daily life around having conscious access to all the states possible for a human, not just the states of being wide awake, stressed, or asleep.

The potential we have in terms of access to different states of consciousness is truly extraordinary, but few people know how to access them, are interested in them, believe they are possible, or are willing to work on them. Hopefully, we can significantly change that on some large level.

The differing states are wonderful to experience as you get good at them. They deeply change your minute-to-minute experience of everything. Many changes stay with you after you do the exercises. It's helpful to learn them with your eyes closed. Later, you can get into methods to use them anywhere at any time; however, the stakes are raised when many things are happening around you that you can hear, see, and smell.

Distractions, attractions, fears, jealousy, external demands, anger, and hatred. These are some of the quickest paths to losing access to more profound states and being able to control your inner environment. None of them are evil; they all have a place in your life. But when you live with them, often you lose the ability to really access the higher states inside you. You'll be pulled powerfully not only into the outer world but also more into the animal and lizard parts of your brain and nervous system. It's very difficult to gain control of your mind, emotions, and energies when you feel like you are on a battlefield. In fact, it's almost impossible.

(By the way it is actually possible to do the exercises in combat and on a battlefield—but you can't *internally* feel like you are on a battlefield and do the exercises. Some martial arts specialize in teaching their students how to do this, but they are rather rare, and that sort of exercise is usually reserved for higher levels of training.)

Questions to help you see what you think and believe about meditative states:

1. What benefits do you think you could receive from working on alternate states of consciousness?
2. What benefits do you think you could receive in your daily life if you could begin to create these states within yourself at will?
3. Do you currently believe that you can't do meditation because it seems hard, or you aren't "good" at it? If so, where did you get that belief from? Have you tried a regular routine at your own pace without expectations of perfection or even general skill at the beginning? (How can you be good at something that you've never tried or practiced before?)

Brain states[6]

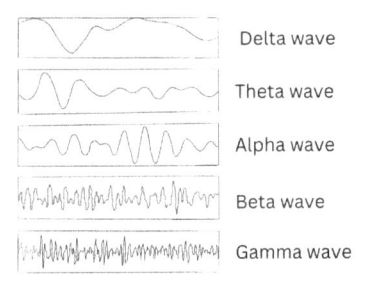

Delta wave

Theta wave

Alpha wave

Beta wave

Gamma wave

Brain waves

I want to give you a brief description of the brain states that are trackable through brain scans.

Beta—this is where most people are during a normal waking state. In high Beta you are stressed, worried, and trying to deal with threats in your environment. High Beta is not a good time to learn or create. Middle and lower Beta are less stressed and are more normal waking states. Most thinking here is linear, logical, spatial, and relies on physical stimulus from the objective world.

Alpha—this state is more relaxed, better for learning, and better for creation. It's meditative, tranquil, and provides enhanced focus. In Alpha you have more of a whole-brain connection and your brain is more suggestible.

Theta—Deep meditation and dreaming sleep are found here. You can experience profound insight, intuition, spiritual connection, creativity, and oneness, if you don't fall asleep here.

Delta—Deep, dreamless sleep and extremely deep meditation lead to Delta. This brain state has a lot to do with rest and repair in your body.

Gamma—In this state, the brainwaves are moving hyperfast. You could rightly call it super-consciousness. It requires methods and practice to reach.

Let me take a minute to describe what the experience of learning the meditative methods that I describe in this book was like for me so I can give you some idea of what they are for and how they change you and your life. Keep in mind this has been a journey of years for me, working and practicing these methods.

When you first try meditation, it's apt to feel like you are herding cats or reining in a wild horse. Your mind will race around. Your emotions will buck at you. Your body will complain. With all those things happening, people usually think they are bad at meditation, contemplation, pranayama, qi gong, and other practices where they have to be still. But that doesn't mean you *are* bad at them—in fact, it means you are starting to work on yourself. That isn't an obstacle, it is actually showing you the path. For me, I intuitively knew that there was an end goal I needed to reach. I could feel it somehow.

Even as a young kid in my backyard, I knew that goal was there and I could reach it. But it took me a long time—and lots of time being led away from it by society—to figure out how to access it regularly and at will. It is a bit of a tricky thing to find in yourself because it is essentially receptive and is found in the quiet. It means reversing the flow of your senses and allowing your mind to slowly rest. Your mind isn't used to resting and the lizard and animal portions of your nervous system are so used to being in overdrive that they perturb your mind to get you into action. They feel safe in your routines and habits. "Worry about this now." "Be angry about this now." "Freak out about the government now." "Panic about getting to work on time now." "Feel anxious about money now." And when you go to gain some control over these automatic behaviors, you'll have to break the loops and cycles.

It isn't that you are bad at it. Rather, it's the base work of gaining some conscious power over unconscious programs in your mind, body, and emotions, and the lizard and animal portions of you will thank you for it. They will begin to feel calm, at peace, and taken care of when your higher functions begin to be present and in control. Your whole system will begin to relax and let go of old routines as you practice and go forward. But for a while, you will be…uncomfortable.

You are supposed to be—otherwise you would miss the opportunity to regulate the old programs and habits. But over time, with a regular relaxed and calm practice of the right methods, it will all calm down within you and the opposite will begin to happen. Everything within you will become quiet. You can reach a point where your mind is calm and unperturbed. Perhaps when you first hear this it sounds boring and weird, but when it happens, you begin to realize your emotions, mind, and body have been in such an uproar your whole life that you have constantly been creating a lot of pain for yourself. You have unconsciously been creating a lot of friction inside, and when it subsides you feel really good, energized, and joyful.

At first this won't occur as ecstasy or bliss, but it is definitely a gentle sort of pretty good feeling. Life begins to feel okay from the inside out. Your mind begins to calm. Your emotions become more settled and less jumpy. Your mind, body, and emotions start to feel like they are something you have and not something you are. And this change is very helpful. Your mind, body, and emotions begin to control you less and less and you begin to have more and more control over them. This makes your experience of life much more pleasant and sweet. Your own mind, emotions, and body can feel like a torture chamber when they are controlling you.

This change can take some time. A lot of things in your body have to change—you are, in a sense, rewiring yourself, and there are bound to be some bumps along the way. But with the right methods, it can go quite quickly. Some methods work much faster than others. And some methods I've learned over time did nothing at all for me. The methods you use matter a lot as does the instruction, but ultimately, you can do all of this, even if you have to find your own way to it. I've tried hard to lay out the best methods possible, and I have hundreds of them that work in different ways that I will teach over time.

At first, meditation might feel like finding your way in the dark. But over time and through practice, you can gain more and more ability over yourself, not in a brutal and domineering way but in a calm, nurturing, growing, and loving way. This can change your entire life from the inside out.

At first you begin to feel everything in your life beginning to get quiet and to fade from your experience. Depending on how chaotic or emotional you were before you started the practice, the time it takes to get to that state will vary, but if you practice regularly, it usually happens rather quickly. The distance traveled becomes smaller and the route is more and more familiar.

As things become quieter and your inner world begins to fill your attention, you sense a feeling of relief and of being uplifted. Thoughts become somehow bigger in your attention. When I first started meditating it was hard to get past this stage. Thoughts are demanding and we often think we are our thoughts. But if you keep practicing and focusing on the techniques over time, the feelings of relief, of being uplifted, and of joy begin to take over the field of consciousness. Then your heart begins to swell in a slow but beautiful way. It swells with a kind of love, but, in fact, you actually experience something physical in your heart as the oxytocin[7] release creates changes in your chemistry and your heart vessels. Body, mind, emotions, and energy are all layered together. Making changes to one affects all the rest.

At this stage, the energy begins to move up your system toward your brain. You can feel the restrictions within your system loosen and the changes in your body, mind, and emotions lifting you up and up. You begin to feel more and more kinds of emotional rushes as you work through the methods. You experience more and more powerful and beautiful emotions. The energies you begin to feel explode and enlighten you. Your mind—your thoughts and imagination—are quiet at this point and you realize that your inner world is much, much bigger than you thought. There is more to you than you could see while your mind was talking or flashing images or stuck in memory or imagination.

This opens you up to past fears and guilt and shame because your ego melts away for a while. You take off the series of masks you always wear. Now, you might notice here that my language gets more and more almost mystical as I describe the experiences. This is because as you go deeper, you go beyond the normal bonds of how you experience yourself and on to something quite a bit greater, more alive, more joyful. The experience of everything changes in color, timing, emotion, thought, and in the opening of intuition and connection. You begin to "hear" more of the greater part of you.

It's quite wonderful at this stage, and you can keep going. The higher and higher you climb—or the more and more refined you go—the more you begin to reach these emotional and energetic peaks of bliss. Then you can explode into ecstasy. In this state, every aspect of you has come to a peak. Your emotions, your focus of attention, your crescendo energies, and your mind are peaking—but quietly. And it all explodes into a nebula of experience within you as you become absorbed into magnificent states of awareness and universal feelings.

When you go through these methods, it takes some time to build the ladder up to reach these experiences within yourself. But because you've trained your mind, emotions, body, energies, and consciousness, you bring some of your normal everyday consciousness with you as you build the ladder. The greatest part of that is that you can consciously hold on to some of it and bring it back into daily life with you without damaging the extraordinary system that you have as a human. It takes longer than blasting through things in a hurry like many try to do. But it ultimately becomes part of you consciously, without any diminishment of your other states of consciousness.

For me, this was all far beyond anything I could have imagined possible for a human being before I experienced it. Nothing else really compares. It is a higher-level aspiration and a more long-term realization than the practices I cover in the Nytality Method, but it may be something you'll find worthwhile working toward, so I mention it here. It can't and won't happen without you moving yourself toward it. You have to expand yourself consciously in your awareness toward it.

But what many people want is to feel better *now*. They want to overcome being stuck in the wake of trauma and feeling worthless or broken. They want to break free of poor health, lack of energy, feeling out of control in their life. Meditation and working with brain states helped me do all of that, which is not to say I am a finished, polished product—that would be just foolishness and a negation of life's evolution. But this work definitely changed me and my life and continues to do so over minutes, days, months, and years. It is a form of treasure that I hope to pass on to you so that you can do the same through your own effort in your own life.

I actually wrote this section after doing some of the exercises I describe in this chapter. Now, I need to come down a bit to go to work. I can't go to work beaming this happily—it can hurt a client who is suffering inside to see someone so up and full of life. So, to paraphrase an ancient saying, I "wear rough clothing and hide the jewel in my heart." I still have it within me, and I still quietly transmit it, but I don't rub it in anyone's face.

Everyone is on their own journey and playing their own role—that is between them and life. You take care of your own piece of life and your own connection to it, that is the best way to be of service. But I still get to carry a lot of that experience within me everywhere I go, and I can always touch back into it on some level. It's wonderful and extraordinary.

Okay, let's take the next step in our journey with these methods.

TEN

CASCADING JOINT MEDITATIONS

THESE METHODS WORK SIMILARLY TO the ones that we've done before. We will be willing our attention through certain parts of our body to create an effect.

1. Sit somewhere comfortable. Sense the top of your head being held up by a string suspended from the ceiling, gently lifting your entire spine.
2. Direct your attention toward your shoulders, both sides at once. Run your attention through your shoulder and into the joint.
3. Move your attention down to your elbows and into the center of the joint until it feels like you are done there. Don't force it, don't try to do it perfectly, don't get lost in the anatomical structure. Play with it and have some fun with it and try to feel everything in the joint as you run your mind to its center.
4. Move down to your wrists. Going from outside to inside will draw your attention into the center of your wrists. It's an interesting act to move your mind to quiet down and relearn how to feel at a deeper level. This will change your use of attention and ultimately your consciousness over time.

5. Move on through your hands, wrist side down, and toward the fingers, paying special attention to each of the knuckles. Take your time going through the hands—there's a lot going on as there are many joints to work through. Have some fun with it. It might be helpful at first to go finger by finger, later you can do them all collectively. Try to be thorough and not miss anything with your mind and attention. Feel it all.

6. Move your attention to your hip joints and playfully draw your attention from the outside to the inside of the joint, starting superficially and going deep. These joints are bigger so there's more for your mind to play with in order to get a good feeling from what you are doing.

7. Draw your attention to your knees and cover as much of each knee as you can, going from the outside to the inside as deep into the joint as you can. When it feels complete, you're done. Don't let your analytical judgment take over because that will make you lose the effect that we're trying to create with these meditative processes.

8. Move down to your ankles, feeling the bones (malleoli) on either side. Start there and move your way deep into the joints, playfully experiencing them until you reach the centers. Let go of everything else as you do this. Nothing else exists at this moment but your ankles.

9. Finally, we get to the feet. Starting at the ankles, draw your attention down through your heels and into the rest of your foot, feeling as much of the foot as you can. Pay special attention as you move into the toe joints and finally work toward the tips of your toes and toenails. Make it fun, make it playful, nothing serious, just something that's useful for every part of you.

10. Now take a few minutes to check how you feel. Focusing your attention on how you feel will help keep your mind calm until you're ready to move back into your day and crush your life.

How to practice the Cascading Joints Meditations:

1. Practice this method for several weeks before lying down in bed to sleep. See if it helps your mind unwind into a more peaceful state.
2. Try doing the Cascading Joints Meditations during the day when you are stressed and need to access another inner state.

ELEVEN

THE WHY OF CHANGING STATE (REACHING YOUR INNER WORLD)

WHY IS CHANGING BRAIN STATE, directing attention, and reaching meditative competence so important? Because all of this is the doorway to your inner state and how you experience what's going on inside you. It changes how your brain processes the information coming into you from outside. It is the doorway and the filter by which you mold and process the information you experience. It is also one of the chief means of being able to conduct your emotions in a way that is beneficial for you and your life.

What you focus your attention on and the brain state you are in determines a massive amount of what you perceive. What you perceive is ultimately the whole picture you take in. If you can alter the picture through your own efforts, you change your whole world.

For some reason this concept can be hard for me to get across to clients, that changing your interface with reality can block you from creating a good life. People have the idea that if you change yourself inside it will keep you from making efforts on the outside to gain a better life. And on some level, this is true: when you can control your inner environment to make you feel okay, you no longer need to control everything outside. You're going directly to the source.

But often it goes beyond that because when you can regulate yourself inside, you get better at changing your life, your environment, and the world around you. Because you're no longer trying to control the uncontrollable, you zero in on what you can actually control. Many people live in a kind of delusion that they can control everyone else, and by doing so they cheat themselves of being able to control much of what they actually can—especially inside.

People spend thousands of hours watching news related to events they literally have no control over, but they ignore studying themselves, their life, and methods for changing their life. They know more about what's happening in a village across the world than they do about what is going on within them—their thoughts, emotions, or body. Some of this, of course, is the natural lizard and animal part of you taking over the human and higher possibilities part of you. These parts of you lack perspective: scale, time, distance, proximity, and so on. They are tuned to seeing everything as a threat. You have to wake up the human and higher possibilities part of you to quiet those impulses, otherwise, you will always be stuck in the lower aspects. You'll basically be an animal. That is a very intense statement that ruffles my feathers, but ultimately it is true. If you let the lizard and animal parts of you rule you, you will be stuck like a slightly higher functioning animal and will never assess your coolest and most evolved parts.

My meditative methods help you recognize and reclaim those aspects of yourself, and they are very helpful in getting you off the "battlefield" in your life so you can move into the "higher" parts of yourself. When you are stuck on the battlefield, your lizard and animal parts tend to take over to keep you safe unless they know that your higher parts are on the job and can handle it. This requires new ways of doing things. It requires that you rewire yourself and reorganize how you function inside. But that reorganization and rewiring will benefit you in hundreds of ways.

Now, let's go back to the example of the news. If you have your attention, mind, and emotions on the news all the time you will always be in a kind of emergency mode. News programming does not show good news. It purposely finds and delivers bad, dangerous, infuriating, and emotional news. You can't live there with your attention and feel good. You can't spend hours there and keep yourself out of animal and lizard dominance.

It's important to know some of what is going on in the world, but I bet if you were truly honest with yourself, you'd realize you can get all of what you need to know in less than 10 minutes a day. The rest is you getting other people's editorializing. It's a form of entertainment that keeps you from accessing the greatest parts of you. You can't create an environment in your head and heart that is always a stressful, chaotic, dangerous battlefield and hope to access all the higher

parts of you consciously and repeatedly. You are working against yourself.

High level martial arts work teaches you how to stay calm in stressful situations to keep the higher parts of you accessible. They specialize in it. They know that if someone can keep you in lizard and animal mode, you are controllable. They actually specialize in keeping you in that mode during conflict so they can purposefully and predictably control you—leading you to your destruction. These animal and lizard parts of you are very powerful and important. You can't suppress or ignore them, and it would be terrible for you if you could. Their power needs to be part of the whole. You need their primal power and even savagery at times. But they need to be put in the proper place within you. That allows you to reclaim the higher and more evolved part of you that makes you human and even more than human.

That's why it's important to learn to change your state inside. Meditative methods, awareness practices, and all the exercises within the Nytality Method are aimed to help you do that. The methods in this book are directly aimed at giving you power over the animal and lizard parts of you that are ruling your body and experience. They are wonderful keys for unlocking your own nervous system, brain states, and reactions to life.

A huge part of this is wisely directing your attention. All the time. The practice of directed attention is a treasure chest for changing your life.

Important questions:

1. Where is your attention going?
2. Where are you shining the light of your consciousness?
3. Are you yourself directing it or is someone else controlling this most valuable asset of yours?

TWELVE

ATTENTION

I'D LIKE TO SPEND SOME more time illuminating why the conscious use of attention is so important. Let's start by looking at a training methodology I kept seeing over and over again while researching ancient and modern methods for self-development.

Student A: "What should I do first to get started on this path, master?"

Master: "Go to the market and get a candle and a rose quickly and then come back."

Student A thinks: "Why am I wasting my time on this? I came here to learn martial arts or yoga."

Student A goes to the market and gets what is required. The owner of the market says, "Oh, you must be a student of the master. He/she has interesting training methods that work in ways you can't yet understand. Heed his/her training or you will miss the essence of what you are."

Student A is perplexed but respectfully thanks the market owner while thinking, "What buffoonery is this? I want to punch someone in the face." Or maybe something like, "I know better than them, they are just giving me busy work. They don't want to give away their secrets. But everyone trusts them, and I saw for myself that the master is somehow… special and different. Plus, Mom and Dad taught me to respect my elders. I had better run back!"

At the same time, the master takes a minute away from resting in union with life and thinks, "I hope this student gets it. Everyone misses the important stuff for tricks, power over others, siddhis (unusual abilities), and their ego. I want to teach everything I know. I hope this one gets it."

The student makes it back to the master and presents what he/she bought. The master looks at the items and is satisfied and can see the perplexed look on the student's face.

"Why the look? What is on your mind and toying with your emotions?" The master asks patiently (hopefully patiently though some versions of the story say "with extreme displeasure").

"It seemed crazy to me to go get these things at the beginning of my instruction. But then the owner of the market said some interesting things to me. He told me people usually miss the

importance of these beginning methods and that I should heed your training. And it knocked some sense in me," says Student A.

"Most people do think that when I send them to get something unexpected. But to get unexpected results you must do unexpected things. The shop owner is an old friend of mine. He knows well the importance of my training as he saw the changes it made in me since our childhood. You are wise to listen to what he said," explained the wise teacher.

The student beamed with the compliment and was glad he/she caught themselves before making a mistake.

The teacher expounds upon the training methods with the candle and rose.

"Every day this month without fail, I want you to spend 15 minutes in this meditation posture with your back straight and looking at the rose. Every time your attention wanders, or your mind starts to run,

or your body starts to complain, and you lose the rose in your perception, bring your attention back to the rose. Admire the rose. Look at its beauty. Admire how beautiful the red color is. As it ages over the days, observe how it breaks down and changes color and eventually gives itself over to the processes of life. Remember to always bring your attention back. Keep the rose in your focused consciousness."

"The candle is equally important. But you will use it at night in the dark, every day without fail for a month. The candlelight will be your beacon in the darkness. It will help you to understand the illumination you are learning with these methods. In the same way as the rose, watch the candle for 15 minutes every night. Watch how it slowly burns down over the nights. Admire its light and the beauty it shines forth. Admire how it illuminates everything around it by shining. Its own success in shining shows everyone around it the way. Every time your mind wants to distract you, bring your attention back to the beautiful candle. Every time your body snarks at you, bring your body back in line. Every time your emotions throw a temper tantrum, calmly let them go and bring your attention back to the candle and its light. Without this training and its diligent practice, you will miss 90% of the training. Your direct attention will determine the rest of your life. It is the drawbridge between you and the outer world. You need to be able to close it and open it at will or the forces outside will overrun your castle and world. Then you will be enslaved. Okay, off you go. Practice these methods, practice them," elucidated the enlightened master.

I found this type of story everywhere as I read in sources from all around the world. Often it was a rose or candle. Other times it would be the moon. The importance of directing your attention consciously through your own efforts is suggested in the story. This is my own adaptation, and I loaded a few other lessons into it to make the most of the story. Some information is best presented in forms that talk to the nonlinear, non-rational, non-obvious parts of your mind. They give birth to understandings well beyond that which a simple obvious breakdown of the idea or principle gives. In modern times, people tend to dislike this approach. They often don't realize their mind is bigger, more powerful, and broader than they know or know how to use.

Partly, teaching in this story form is in itself a teaching on how to reclaim those aspects of yourself and your mind. It also uses your emotions and feelings to help convey ideas and understandings and helps lock the information in your mind. The story form itself is a memorization instruction. It teaches some important understandings of how your memory works. For example, your memory likes stories, and it builds on similarity. It causes powerful connections in your mind and builds bigger connections in your brain.

Attention is one of your most important assets along with time and health. In fact, it may actually be impossible to separate yourself from your attention. Without attention you really don't exist. If you have ever been knocked out in surgery, you have experienced this. Your body still exists in the material world but are you still there? Are you experiencing anything at all? Your consciousness at that point is ultimately concealed. In the case of surgery, mercifully concealed.

But the experience is gone. Your attention is the fundamental resource you have to experience life.

Choose how you experience your life. Consciously choose where you put your attention. Everything else depends on it.

Start to play with changing where you put your attention and notice the change in how you feel. That's the key to learning what's happening within you. It starts with where you put your attention. For example, if you put your attention on things that upset you for long periods of time and those are things you can't do anything about, how do you feel afterward?

Questions for your attention!
(Exclamation points get your attention)

1. How do you feel if you consciously direct your attention to something you find beautiful and uplifting?
2. Can you find places to focus your attention that help you feel better and more full of vitality?
3. Can you consciously pull your attention away from areas that don't serve you but rather scare you or give you anxiety?

THIRTEEN

THE ACTIVATING METHODS

A FEW YEARS AGO, ONE of my long-time clients—we'll call him Tom although that's not his real name—texted me after he had a terrible head injury. He indicated he was struggling with its after-effects.

The aftereffects of a traumatic brain injury (TBI) can be devastating in multiple ways. Recovery can be difficult and rarely do people know what to expect. That goes not only for the person who suffered the head injury but for the people around them too.

For the person with a TBI, their ability to perceive what is going on around them can be considerably reduced. Their ability to function emotionally can shift. They can have a hard time with recall of memories, and they may have a significant change in their personality. From my experience, these are just a few of the changes that can come from a TBI.

This is, of course, tough for the person who suffered the injury. But it's also hard for the people in their life because the symptoms can make the person with the TBI seem like a different person than the one they knew before the injury.

Tom had all the symptoms I mentioned above, plus migraines and other kinds of headaches. He was reading everything he could find about recovering from the injury but wasn't finding the solutions he needed. He was, he said, almost at the point of giving up. Tom asked if I could help.

I spent a few months working with him on a number of my methods and in time Tom showed remarkable improvement. During one of the last times I saw him for his TBI problems, he made a very concerted effort to tell me how much my methods had helped him. He implied they had saved his life figuratively and literally.

Every once in a while, a client says something that almost brings me to tears, and this was one of those moments. He also urged me to teach as many people as possible the methods that I have made.

It can be easy to think there is nothing that can be done for certain problems. But no matter what problem you're experiencing, I implore you to keep seeking answers. They may not be in the first place you look, or even the 50th, but you would be surprised at what is possible when you remain resolute in your search for solutions.

So, let's begin working on some really important methods that are unique, so far as I have been able to discover in my research on this system. I would be surprised if other people don't have something similar in their work but for me these methods were inspired by a desperate need to

get my brain and nervous system to heal from long-term infections that damaged my health. I spent years and I'm sure literally thousands of hours of study to compile the context and

understandings needed to make this healing process work within myself. But work within me it definitely has. It has widely and deeply changed every aspect of my life.

I really had no idea how sick and how far off I was because I got sick so young, and the intense trauma on top made it even more confusing and hard to see. In addition, my ability to perceive, think, and remember was impaired, making it almost impossible for me to see what was going on until the healing itself showed up for me. I don't much like talking about sickness, disease, trauma. I know that the mind is an extraordinarily powerful creation machine, so I don't think it's wise to put a lot of attention on these sad aspects of life. But sometimes they create understanding and context that's important for connecting the dots. So, I want to take a little time here to expand on what happened in what now seems like a past life for me.

I really couldn't understand how slowly my mind was processing and how much difficulty I was having in connecting concepts. I also didn't realize how much my perception was shifting, depending on my energy levels and health. On some level, some part of me knew that, and that created a fair amount of anxiety and frustration. It's amazing to watch your mind go from an average computer down to a calculator, and then up to a supercomputer because everything changes within you. It's a truly surreal and painful experience but one that ultimately taught me that I am not my mind. It really helps to separate my consciousness from my mind in my experience. Honestly, that understanding is worth its weight in gold although this isn't the only way to get it. I couldn't even commiserate with anyone because I didn't know anyone who had been through similar things. And I am grateful for that. I don't wish those things on anyone.

But the techniques I describe in this book helped me more than anything else I did for myself or with doctors for the specific problems that I am describing here. I did get a lot of help from different doctors, an acupuncturist, and therapists but my own techniques really helped my brain and mind get over my main difficulties.

The work needs to be done in the right order and together in the right package to achieve the desired effect. It took me an enormous amount of experimentation, long trial and error, research, and playing with that balance until it created a cascade that changed everything for me in this specific area with my brain, mind, and emotions. I have hundreds of other methods which have helped me in innumerable ways, but this method gave me the keys to heal what I assume were problems with my central nervous system in truly unexpected and hard to describe ways. The way I now personally apply these methods is rather comprehensive and complex. I will teach the whole thing, but for this book I cut it down into something manageable and memorizable but still extraordinarily effective.

I didn't figure everything out at once but rather in chunks and in pieces. I'll present a more refined and shortened version for you to use than the one I followed. I would be somewhat devastated if there were someone like me who desperately needed this information but who wasn't able to use it because it looked too long and daunting.

While I do believe steps need to be done in a certain order, you don't need to do them all at once. Please be careful not to force these; I have knocked myself on my ass overdoing them, and though I never had any long-term ill effects, it certainly wiped me out for a while. I believe the methods in this book to be extremely safe as the changes and effects derive from self-healing and self-building processes. The process is like removing blockages and getting the right resources (oxygen, blood flow, nerve signals from point A to point B, for example) to get things done.

The specific methods in this section rely in particular on the idea of getting signals in your nervous system from point A to point B. This has a powerful effect on all kinds of functions in your system. This was surprising to me. I have specialized my somatic therapy work in focusing on the possibilities of using the interconnectedness of the body, mind, emotions, and energies within a human—yet even so, I was shocked by the massive, immediate, and obvious changes this made in my system. It still blows my mind reflecting back on it. Who would have guessed that working on yourself inside could change you so much? I only had my intuition about it but I'm grateful I listened to it and followed it to these conclusions.

I do want to make a strong point here that these techniques not only helped my healing and recovery but have also taken me well beyond what I expected was possible. They have been wonderfully powerful in changing my state, changing my mood, inspiring thought and mental connections, clearing fatigue, and calming me down after stressful situations. I could go on, but I'll leave you to experience them for yourself.

These techniques can be done sitting, walking, or lying down once you get the hang of them, and as long as you don't have something you need to pay attention to like driving a car or operating heavy machinery. I personally wouldn't go anywhere near these techniques while drinking or doing drugs. I don't think I would try these while involved with any recreational psychoactive substances. Some of the exercises involve working with your neurotransmitters and you won't have any idea what results you are getting because you will be spiking and then depriving your body of specific neurotransmitters and certain important trace chemistry if you are doing any psychoactive drugs. That's how the drugs work, they change the same chemistry we want to impact inside with these methods. So, tread carefully. I'm not trying to harsh your mellow and I'm not trying to reinforce old stereotypes with this. I don't know what would happen and I wouldn't be willing to play with my brain to find out. Chances are you would just lose the ability to get anything done with these methods, but brain chemistry is very, very specific and I wouldn't risk it. All right, that's the warning. ⚠

So, let's start by sitting up straight. It matters that your spine is straight and that you aren't tense. Don't get fanatical about it, but it does make a difference. Laser focus is also crucial for these techniques to work in the beginning as it helps to have clear intention, understanding, and sustainable attention. I've been trying to build some understanding of these faculties throughout the book but let me take a minute to describe what I mean here by clear intention.

Clear intention is knowing specifically, consciously, and without any confusion what you are trying to do, and then holding that in your mind while you perform what you are doing. A lot of the "holding in your mind" is done in your subconscious mind. You plant the seed clearly and directly and that will help the deep parts of your mind work. You tell those deep parts of your mind what is to be done specifically and clearly. That is as crucial for these methods as it is for many other areas of life.

Try to practice the exercises in a place where you won't be disturbed or distracted. It's really tough to do these with lots of distractions. Ultimately, this is a journey deep inside you, exploring how you are wired and how you work through experience and feeling. It reconnects to what your body knows, what your feeling sense knows, what the animal and lizard parts of you know, what you knew before your analytical mind got so busy with abstraction, imagining the future, remembering and analyzing the past—taking you completely out of your body, out of your feelings, out of your here, and out of your now.

We are working on building an owner's manual in your experience that you can use. Nothing will happen if you just read the information in this book. Nothing will happen if you just memorize how these are done. Nothing will happen if you just read this and judge it. We spend so much time in school being told what to look at. We memorize it for tests. We judge and criticize it.

It's very easy to confuse memorizing and knowing the names of things with true understanding. That's how educational models function, and to be fair it's not that easy to create situations for everything to be done in a classroom setting—and to learn properly. It's hard to test what students actually know. This isn't meant to be a frontal attack on the current educational model, but it is a fact that deserves some elucidation here.

When I was teaching at a junior college, I kept tripping over this with my students. I would be teaching an anatomy class and some students would be upset when I would have them feel their own tibia or the manubrium of their partners. They were so used to just looking at pictures, it really bugged a few of them when I encouraged them to actually apply the knowledge to gain understanding. Most loved it, they were excited and almost thirsty to do something with what they were learning. Some people really do love thinking and abstract thinking specifically. I am definitely one of them. Maybe you can tell by how I write and are laughing at the pot calling the kettle black. I know one of my weaknesses lies in doing physical things. The trick is to know where your strengths and weaknesses lie.

In one of the ancient traditions I studied as a kid, they spoke at length about three kinds of people. They said everyone thinks they see the world the same but there is a fundamental difference in how they perceive it. Some people perceive and relate to the world mostly through their body, some mostly through their mind, and some mostly through their emotions. Of course, there are admixtures of all three in every person. Some people are hyperstrong in one area and weak in the other two. Some are kind of strong in two and weak in one. The narcissist thinks they are equally good at all three. They would say that one of the great goals in life is to get all three working well within you and together with each other. That usually means taking a break from where you are strongest—or actually taking attention and time away from it to work on the area/s where you are weak. If one of the areas seems stupid to you, that is the area to work on. A lot of people—doers—will mock heavy thinkers for example. A lot of mind people, deep-thinking types, will mock the emotions and see them as a waste and something that requires no attention or active suppression. A lot of emotional types, often really creative, will ignore their mind and body and might even get lost in drug use, ignoring the damage it may cause the mind and body.

Of course, this is all subjective, but I have found profound truth in this idea and my understanding of people and in relationships. People will be in heated arguments because they aren't speaking the same language through the same perspective and so they can't come to any accord or melding of the mind, heart, and body. They won't be able to see the other's perspective unless they understand that they are coming from very different perspectives. People tend to think that others think like they do. It could be quite an interesting awakening to realize that people might have distinctly different vantage points.

For example, a very cerebral person might want to talk about concepts and philosophies, but their significant other might be very physical and far more interested in cuddling, hiking, sex, and physical proximity with one another. You might think of these as aspects of personality and of course some of that is true, but I do believe some of it is deeper within you and connected to how you are wired. That doesn't mean two opposite types can't do well with each other; they can absolutely help each other grow and evolve. On the other hand, two people of the same type in temperament might find it really easy to be together but find that they don't necessarily feel the same evolution and growth that could be thrilling for them.

There are lots of possibilities here depending on what you want and what kind of relationships you prefer. But the most important relationship in this regard is you with yourself. How do you function in this regard? What is your greatest strength? Where is your weakness? Do you have two obvious weaknesses? If you feel like you have no strength, then you're probably way too hard on yourself. Everyone has a strength and it's important to recognize that in yourself. If you were to consider a continuum between self-degradation and arrogance, then humility (a word that crops up frequently in translations of ancient teachings) actually sits in the middle of the continuum. Humility isn't hating yourself or attacking yourself mentally and emotionally. This point seems hard for people to grasp, I know many super arrogant people who think that they are humble, and I know many self-hating and self-deprecating people who think they are just being humble. For some reason, it really isn't that easy to see humility in yourself.

I wanted to take a minute to explain all this to hopefully help you see that not everyone has the same viewpoint and vantage point. Not everyone is built the same, so don't beat up on yourself or others. The Nytality Method absolutely requires all three aspects of yourself, you need to understand the concepts, practice them, and work them into your life and feel the results. Ideally, you'll feel the results in both a physical sense and an emotional sense, otherwise, you won't experience the full result—if any at all—from these methods. But please make sure that you practice them. Nothing will happen without the doing itself.

I want to mention that some traditions break this down into four types rather than three, so along with the physical person, the mental person, and the emotional person, you also have the energy person. The energy person is very interested in the energy within themselves and in life. I personally think that using the four differentiations is closer to the truth, but for Western audiences this can be a little confusing since we don't talk about energy in the same way and with the same perspective. I'll leave it in your hands to decide for yourself. You might indeed think that all people are exactly the same and that this is all BS with no relevance to you or your life, in which case just throw these concepts and understandings away and go on with what works for you. None of this matters if you can't make it work for you in your life in some way.

This is your project, your life, your lab, your education, your experience—it is all about the real authentic you.

Practices and questions to apply in your life right now:

1. Watch yourself for a month and write down what is mostly in your attention. What is usually going on in your emotions, your mind, and your body?
2. You probably think that you know what's going on within your mind, emotions, body, and energy levels. But most people really don't: it all

happens automatically and mostly without much attention. Try to watch yourself. Is most of your attention and focus on mental and intellectual things? Is it on creative pursuits: music, art, emotions, and empathy for others? Is it mostly exercise with your body? Do you love being in the gym? Do you make the most progress by taking lots of action or by planning well and then acting on the plan?

3. In which areas are you the weakest? Which areas do you try to avoid? Do you hate to work out? Do you dislike thinking deeply on subjects? (Don't mistake worry and anxiety pushing your mind in directions as thinking deeply.) Do you see music, art, emotions, and personal relationships as a waste of time?

FOURTEEN

THE ACTIVATING METHODS

OKAY, LET'S GET TO IT. We will start this work sitting on the floor or on a chair, just make sure your spine is reasonably straight and without much stressful pressure on it. Lift your head, feeling a little light pull toward the ceiling.

The following methods are done to activate an effect on specific nervous system areas and glandular centers in a sequential pattern. We are looking to create nerve-signal traffic from point A to point B while simultaneously creating a change in our brain states from Beta to Alpha and on through the other brain states all the way to Gamma. This is a bit of a fancy way to say that we are trying to make a cascading impact on your nervous system and your glands that will help your body function better in these areas. While it moves you into different brain states so that you feel different inside, what is key is that it helps you—through your own efforts—to feel better inside. This is my experience of what is going on inside me with these methods, and it really makes a big change in how I function during the day. This also describes what it feels like to do the exercises correctly.

Step 1

We will start with the lumbosacral nerve plexus,[8] a web of nerves in the lumbar and sacral region of the body. It sits on the front side of your lower back and goes through your pelvis and down into your legs.

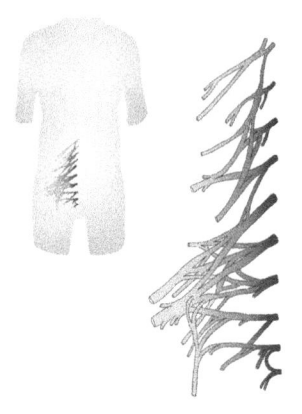

Lumbosacral nerve plexus

You only need to know approximately where this is in your body. You don't need to become an anatomist or go to any dissections. You just need a general idea so that you can direct your attention to it and try to reconnect to the part of you that can feel it. Your nervous system obviously knows exactly where it is and knows the path between your brain and this plexus. This is all about putting your attention there and then holding it there for a few moments until it feels as though your attention has "activated it." All that means is that you feel like you've awakened your nervous system by directing your attention and mind at the structure. In this case, at the lumbosacral plexus.

So, after you sit down, relax, straighten your spine, and feel like your head is suspended from the ceiling or even the sky or a star above. Pull your attention from the top of your head down to the lumbosacral plexus, then rest your attention there. Leave it there for up to a minute. For now, there isn't any reason to stay there longer than a minute. This is about actively relaxing and recovering peace within yourself. Don't force it. That being said, if you feel drawn to stay on this structure for a while, by all means follow the feeling and let it guide you. Play with this and don't force it to work. Make it specific but not hard work.

Really milk the feeling where you think the plexus is. Your attention and mind will zero in on the place over time as the subconscious mind recognizes what you are trying to do. You aren't creating a picture or map in your head with this. The picture and map already exist in the most intricate and perfect version, well beyond anything your conscious mind and imagination can build. Just tune back into it consciously and playfully. Heavy-duty thought, imagination, or remembering a picture in a book will block the feeling and you won't get nearly as much done.

This is step one of the activating method. Honestly, it's as easy as it seems—the work is done by the conscious reconnection itself. Directing your attention, your conscious mind, your subconscious mind, your feeling senses, and your physical senses toward this one area of your body will do interesting things as you practice it over time. You can do each anatomical structure three times in a row and/or three times throughout the day. I wouldn't do more than that. There is something sort of magical that happens when you do all these methods three times. In fact, in many of the meditation methods I've learned or have read about in disciplines throughout the world, rounds of three are often preferred. It seems to have a powerful effect.

Step 2

The second step, focused on the spine, will be easier to understand as it is more familiar and is easily palpable if you want to feel it.

The spine

In this step we will be working with the entirety of the spine, from the neck down to the sacrum. We will not only use the bone but also everything inside including the meninges, the cerebral spinal fluid, and the spinal cord. The meninges are three levels of dural tissue that sit within the bone and around the spinal cord.

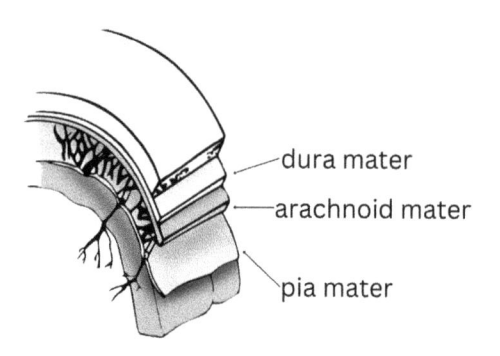

dura mater
arachnoid mater
pia mater

Meninges

The cerebrospinal fluid is a fluid that fills the skull and the spine all the way down to the sacrum. Don't worry too much about understanding these specifics because, again, your mind and body already know everything about your spine, so all you need to do is reconnect. Try to feel and connect your attention to your entire spine in a complete but relaxed and playful way. This isn't work that is meant to be hard but rather work that is meant to be playful and joyful. The manner in which you work matters deeply, not only in these exercises but everywhere in life.

Take your attention away from the top of your head where it has been feeling suspended and draw it down your spine from top to bottom or draw it from bottom to top—whatever you prefer at the moment. Once your attention has been drawn along the spine's length, focus it on your entire spine for up to a minute—usually not longer unless you're really drawn to it. Don't strain, don't struggle—there is no one watching or judging. Don't judge yourself. This is an easygoing exercise and will wake the spine up as you practice it over time.

Again, you can do this once, twice, or three times in a row or during the day, but don't do more than that. You don't want to overdo this.

Have some fun with this and experiment in a playful and beautiful but dutiful way. Reframe how you see work and get something done. We are training ourselves to a whole new mode of accomplishing, work, and action.

Step 3

Okay, in the next step we are going to move on to working with the heart. I think most people have some understanding of what and where their heart is but let's clarify a little bit. Your heart is in your upper chest a little bit left of the centerline just off the sternum and deep to the ribs. It pumps your blood as well as being integral to getting oxygen into the blood from the lungs.

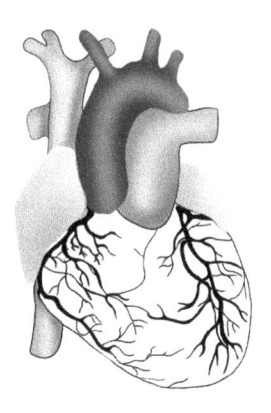

Heart

That part you know. What people often don't know is that your heart also has a large collection of sensory dendrites, generally around 40,000, which act like a small brain. And it's for this reason we want to use it for this exercise.

For me, learning of this nervous system within the heart has effectively changed how I put my work together and how I function. It has also helped my blood pressure. I discussed this collection of nerves at length in my last book, *Ah, Brain, Why Do You Trouble Me So Much?* So, I won't dwell on it here, but it is substantially more important than you might think.

1. Sit somewhere comfortable. Roll your hips slightly forward. Sit up so your spine is mostly straight and lift your head toward the ceiling. Feel that you are lifting with the crown of your head, the very top or where the soft spot was when you were a baby.
2. Take your attention from the top of your head and drive it down to your heart.
3. Move your attention from the outside of your heart to the inside and hold it there for up to a minute unless you feel drawn to stay longer.
4. Take a moment to experience how you feel. Did this work with your heart change your state? Do you feel more energy, or do you feel like you need a nap?

We will get further into this work with the heart later, but for now it's a wonderful place to start. I was surprised by its power when I first started using this exercise. There's a lot more going on with your heart and the nerve plexus within it than is easy to see. Really focus on it and try to feel it.

Going further now, we will start working with the base of your brain where it meets your spinal cord. The brain stem is the posterior part of the brain that connects the cerebrum with the spinal cord. It is composed of the pons, the midbrain, and the medulla oblongata.[9]

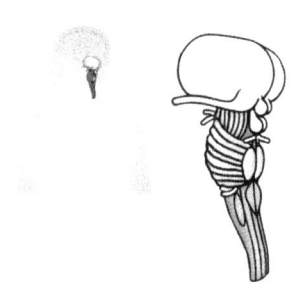

Brain stem

This is the central trunk of the mammalian brain and it's important that we address this area in our work. I will avoid going into depth over anatomy and functions because I want you to focus on just doing the exercise for now. If you think of focusing your work where the top of your spine meets the base of your skull—inside the upper vertebrae and the tissue that goes through the hole at the bottom of your skull—you'll be in the right area for this work.

This particular exercise might take extra attention at first because this area of your body is a little less familiar than, say, your heart or spine, but it is really important that it works right. Even just writing about it is activating a nice effect for me. I had a long day with clients and subtly reconnecting has really lifted my mood and lightened some pressure in my head and neck. I love the impact these exercises have had on me over months of practice in my daily life.

1. Find a warm, comfortable spot and sit either on the floor or on a chair. Roll your hips forward and elongate your spine toward the ceiling.
2. Focus your attention on the top of your head. Feel like you are slightly and pleasantly hanging from the ceiling.
3. Draw your attention from the top of your head to the point at the top of your spine and at the base of your skull inside the bone.
4. Hold your attention there for up to a couple of minutes. I often hold

this position longer because it feels better to do so. But try it out for yourself to see how it feels. Don't force it if it doesn't feel good to hold for a while. The hold is just maintaining your attention in this area to create the desired effect.

5. Take some time to see how you feel afterward. Do you feel differently than before you started? In what way?

Step 4

We will finish this section with one last exercise focused just above where we were in step 3.

The Limbic Brain

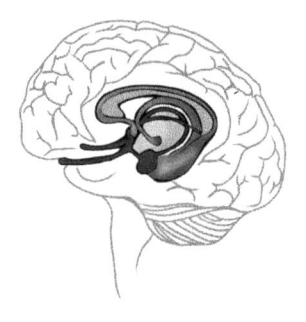

Limbic system

The limbic system,[10] also called the paleomammalian cortex, is a set of brain structures located on both sides of the thalamus, beneath the temporal lobe. It supports a variety of functions including behavior, emotions, and long-term memory. One's emotional life is mostly contained in the limbic system, and it is very important in the creation of memories.

So, if you return to the area where we just had your attention housed and move it toward the center of your brain, you will get to the general area of your limbic system.

This area is very important for lots of deep functions going on within you and it's a wonderfully important area to add to the work that we're doing here. When I learned to activate this specific area, I experienced massive positive changes. Why exactly this works I don't entirely know but there does seem to be something important about sending signals from one part of you to another part of you through where you put your attention, what you are trying to feel, and repeatedly making the connection. It seems to have a wonderful sort of rewiring effect. Just remembering this now and describing it has me feeling a bit high in a way. It's really extraordinary what's possible for a human to do with the right understanding and practice.

1. Sit somewhere comfortable, hips rolled forward and head "suspended" from the ceiling.
2. Focus your attention on the top of your head and then slowly move it down to the limbic system, right above the brain stem and very deep in your brain. (Remember you don't have to be perfect with this. A part of you knows exactly where this is, and you are just consciously reminding yourself where it is on the inside of you.
3. Focus your attention on this deep part of your brain and hold it in that area for up to a couple of minutes. Be careful not to go past what feels comfortable for you right here and right now. It's very important that you tune into yourself and follow the feeling inside. Strain is your enemy.
4. After holding your attention in this area for a sufficient amount of time, let go and just feel. How do you feel right now? How does your body feel? How do you feel emotionally?

These four steps are a wonderful place to start and to practice for a few weeks before moving on to the next section. It's important to get good at each step and section before moving on to the next set so you don't overwhelm your ability to do these comfortably and capably. You have plenty of steps here to make a nice change and to begin understanding and practicing how these methods work. Play with these for a while before you move on to the next part.

We have a lot more to cover in this book and the results build on the strength of the previous exercises being done well. It's like constructing a building: you need to do things sequentially from the foundation up.

But, most important, play with this. Play with it to make it work for you. Don't make it too serious but do follow the instructions.

FIFTEEN

PERSONAL EXPERIENCE OF THE FULL METHOD (WHAT YOU MIGHT EXPECT)

BIOLOGICAL UPGRADE

LOOKING BACK OVER THE DECADES that I've been working with clients, it seems I've come to specialize in working with people suffering from difficult, complex, or undiagnosed problems. This was unintentional, but on closer examination it's not all that surprising. I think my personal history helps me relate to people dealing with these types of problems. I also think the complexity of helping people with these hard-to-pin-down problems keeps my brain engaged.

Often these problems need creative solutions that involve building up the health of a person enough that the problem practically heals itself.

This brings me to a story about my client Caterina. She is in her late twenties, into fitness, and follows a healthy diet, but she was having a myriad of odd symptoms: sleep problems, light depression that comes and goes, malaise, and feeling uninspired. She was also prone to colds and the flu. These kinds of symptoms are common to many ailments, making it hard to pin down their exact source.

Soon after I began working with Caterina, her tendency to catch colds and flu improved greatly but we kept hitting a wall on her problems with her emotions, sleep, and energy level. To help Caterina break through that wall, I began teaching her one of the systems in this book, the Vital Brain Method. She began to practice the first part of the method and after a few weeks, I noticed the energy returning to her eyes. I could also hear it in her voice and see it in her body language. It was as if an invisible cloud that had been following her around like Charlie Brown's rain cloud had finally disappeared.

"There is just something about this brain work you are teaching me," she said. "It's like scratching the deepest itch I can find. I feel 10 to 20% better than I can ever remember feeling. I can't wait to learn the second part of these incredible methods. How in the world did you figure out how to do these?"

"Oh, just a few decades of being obsessed with finding the answer," I said.

Caterina's comments are typical of the feedback I get on these methods. People seem to get a biological upgrade that improves their health, immune system, emotional state, mental capacity, and even how they relate to trauma. They just generally feel better. So, I would like to describe for you what happened when I finally figured out how to combine these methods into a complete package. This will help you understand why I was so excited about them as well as why I give a few warnings to go a little slow and pace yourself. One caveat: I don't believe most people will have anywhere near the same intense changes as I did for two major reasons. Number one, you probably don't have the same infections in your body that I carried around for decades nor the intense trauma that I suffered at the hands of my tormentor. Number two, because I put these methods together, I know exactly how they're meant to work and how they work together, and that magnified the effect that I

PERSONAL EXPERIENCE OF THE FULL METHOD (WHAT YOU MIGHT EXPECT)

felt. I'm presenting this to you in a slower and more controlled fashion. I've already experienced the pain for you, so we can do this in a smarter way.

I had been working on these ideas in a specific way for months. When I reached the point where I figured out the last key element, it was as if, all at once, the door I needed to open was fully opened. I had gotten many small glimpses at my health, thinking processes, emotional stability, and perception but this was a huge pivot point for my life and for my work.

One night I was lying awake working on some ideas related to getting the changes I needed and suddenly a whole set of new concepts, ideas, and methodology blasted into my mind. I've learned over the years that when this happens, I need to get it out of my head as quickly as possible so I don't lose it. After writing it down, I practiced it, and I could feel huge changes come over me. Even afterward I felt quite energetic, peaceful, and relaxed.

A few hours later I noticed something very interesting happening within my body. The roof of my mouth started to ooze mucous. It also began to come out of the sides of my cheeks as well as my upper gums. Then my nose began to bleed for a while and then it also oozed. This knocked me out for a few days where all I could do was go to work and come home and sleep. I figured I probably just had a cold. But a few days later, when I was feeling better, I did the methods again and the same thing happened in the same time frame. But at the same time, my mind felt clearer than ever before and that lasted for several hours. I also felt an interesting release of my tendency toward negative emotions, such as my free-floating anxiety, which had no discernible cause. That was something I had been desperately seeking release from, so it piqued my curiosity.

I waited a few more days to feel better and then did the methods again and I got a similar result with cold or flu-like symptoms. The symptoms reduced this time maybe 10%, but the clear mind, more access to positive emotion, and a general sense of well-being was improved by 10%. By this point I was truly becoming excited to see the potential of these methods in my life.

Again, I waited a few more days and did the exercises again. Just as before, I got a 10% reduction in the flu- and cold-like symptoms and an improvement in everything else. As I kept going, the flu-like symptoms slowly reduced, and the feeling of well-being and clarity improved and improved and improved. I was beside myself with elation and excitement, but I was also worried that these amazing results wouldn't be permanent or replicable. Yet in time I realized the results went deep within my system; there was no going back to the old infections that had plagued me for decades.

I cannot describe how much relief I felt with these improvements. I also felt great satisfaction from having figured a lot of this out through my own dedication, persistence, and research. In many ways I owe my life to my doctor, my acupuncturist, and my therapist. I also owe a great debt to people in the past who wrote down their healing methods, spiritual practices, and personal development work. But ultimately, I also owe myself some appreciation for continuing to pursue what might be possible for me and my health; otherwise I wouldn't be here.

When you have a true treasure, I think the natural impulse is to share it with others. You want to present it in such a way that other people can understand its value and use it in their own life. But with a health and well-being treasure, it's not so easy for many people to see. Many people would rather have $1 million than mental clarity, emotional stability, and even soaring pleasant emotions at will. I know a small handful of millionaires and my guess is that all of them would trade most of that to solve the health problems, mental problems, and emotional problems they face. I know because I have asked them and spent many hours working to help them resolve their problems.

Would you rather have real mental clarity and the ability to think well, or $3 million and a confused and chaotic mind? Of course, in real life the two are not mutually exclusive, I'm just making a point. Would you rather have pleasant and enjoyable emotions, or would you rather have enormous financial wealth?

Let me be clear, I'm not really talking about genuine poverty and starvation. You do need food, water, and shelter. But even in extreme poverty you'd still want a clear, highly functioning mind and an appropriate emotional life. Both of these functions will be extremely useful in pulling yourself out of your current situation which is genuinely dire.

The next benefit of these methods that I'd like to describe is the massive change in my memory. This is interesting to talk about in part because of the current problems with Alzheimer's and other forms of dementia. I do wonder if my methods will have application in the prevention or even perhaps in the treatment of such maladies. But that is well beyond my current purpose here.

At the beginning of my treatments for my infections, my memory—which had never been particularly great—got obviously worse. Over the years, as we killed the infections and worked to heal my body, my memory got better and better to the point that I was remembering things that had totally disappeared for me earlier. It was an extraordinary experience, but it was somewhat limited and fleeting. It would come and go at unexpected times.

The exercises that I describe in this book brought it back tenfold—permanently. I would have moments where I would see a flock of geese fly overhead and instantly remember 10 other experiences that were visually similar, with full sensation—experiences I had completely forgotten about before. There were times that this experience almost knocked me on my ass, recognizing how much I had forgotten previously and how much my memory was changing. It was becoming informational as well as visual.

To describe how this has changed my life is virtually impossible. How do you describe forgetting most of your history and your life and then suddenly having it all come back? How do you describe a change in memory that goes from factual remembering of data to remembering active visual, audial, and sensory detail?

These visual changes also occurred in my comprehensive and analytical mind. Suddenly I could visualize things significantly better and with more detail and with more clarity. It has really shocked me to my core.

Part of the reason I mention this story is because it illustrates something I think affects memory loss. I had been in excruciating pain for decades every single day almost without fail. If I could remember that, as I can now, while I was still experiencing it, it might have driven me crazy. I don't say that to minimize mental health, simply to clarify how important I think it is. My memory now seems to be reasonably eidetic—full of vivid images. That would've made the hell of what I was experiencing tenfold back in the day. In many ways it was a huge blessing that my mind and memory protected me from that fate. Sometimes what seems like a terrible or horrible thing is actually the best thing for you. Then, when you can finally change the situation, you can remove the painful or difficult thing and see the value it held for you at that time.

My memory now is still somewhat up and down. Sometimes I remember everything in perfect, almost excruciating detail and at other times it's just pretty good. It's still improving as I work with the methods in this book as well as other methods within my system. I don't yet know how far the benefits and improvements can go but I'm dang sure going to find out. The methods in this book are wonderful and they fit like pieces of a puzzle that make up the Nytality Method. Each piece individually is quite extraordinary—at least for me—and the whole thing together is radically and wonderfully life-changing in ways I couldn't even begin to imagine before I started putting it together. I don't much like talking about it in these glowing and almost unbelievable terms because I don't want it to sound like snake oil, but how else will you get a sense of it if I don't talk about it at least a little? Right now, I'm alone treading the path for this work, but I want to share it with as many people as I can. I'm leaving a trail of breadcrumbs to where it goes; it is important to me to get people to start walking down the same path.

Another interesting improvement I experienced in doing these methods was an almost complete reduction in long-term neck pain and upper back pain (I think it was from a form of meningitis and/or encephalitis from the infections). However, I imagine the same methods would work for people with other neck, head, or back pain too. The exercises have also helped with my sense perceptions. All my senses have become actively sharper. This has been going on since the middle of my treatment cycles for the infections, but my Nytality work took it to whole new levels of perception and consistency.

Hopefully this gives you some things to think about as well as some inspiration to practice these methods regularly and with focus. Let's move on to a breathing exercise that fits into this overall method: the push breath.

SIXTEEN

THE PUSH BREATH

YOU MIGHT NOTICE THAT SOME of the breathing methods in this book are reasonably active and a little explosive. In these breathing exercises our primary focus is to feel like we are oxygenating the system and then using that oxygenation to work with our nervous system changes. It seems to improve the overall effect.

There was something important for me when I began playing with changing the oxygenation and how my brain was functioning. I have other simple breathing exercises for calming the system down and for making some other cool changes, but the two we have done so far in this book are specifically about ramping the system up a bit and improving gas exchange (carbon dioxide and oxygen). Gas exchange helps the methods get into your system deeper and more profoundly. Later, I'll show you how to interconnect all these methods into a full system to create the largest effect. We are building something step by step and ultimately, we will put it all together in a cohesive pattern that maximizes the connections.

Let's get into this reasonably simple but powerful breathing process. It does a wonderful job of picking you up energetically. I made it to help take the oxygenation feel from the first breath that is pushed inside to the spine and up to the brain into the legs and arms as well. So, with this breath we will pull the air in quickly and then push it out to the extremities. This gets everything moving in your extremities to help the overall circulation. We will layer this into the spine and brain later in the last breathing method, which will help the Activating Methods work.

This one might be best learned lying on your back with your hands on your stomach, but it can be done lying, sitting, or standing.

1. Lie on your back comfortably with your hands on your stomach.
2. Take in a quick, deep breath and try to fill your stomach and then your chest with air.
3. This inhalation can last five to six seconds. It's not slow but rather quick and energetic.
4. Push the air into your arms and legs, leading it with your mind but also by contracting the muscles in your torso.
5. Push the exhalation out of your mouth and nose while you push the air to your arms and legs and down to your hands and feet.
6. While doing the push, contract your belly into your spine and then push up the belly and diaphragm toward your head—a light vacuum contraction. This will help with feeling the push of air into your arms and legs and will also help stimulate the vagus nerve, which has a huge impact on your system and energizes your organs.
7. The vacuum in the preceding breath will stimulate the next breaths into a nice in and out cadence as you practice this breathing exercise. Ten breaths in and out seem to be ideal to get something powerful done without stressing and straining yourself.
8. When you finish your breathing sequence, take a few minutes to check how you feel. For me, this breathing is quite invigorating and lifts me up when I'm a bit tired. It's also surprisingly good at helping with cold hands and feet.

🔖 **NOTE:** When first practicing this exercise, it's helpful to have your hands on your stomach so you can feel the inhalation and exhalation: how much you're drawing into your belly and how much you push out and vacuum. This gives you immediate, palpable, and tangible feedback on what you were trying to accomplish. Learning these methods while lying on your back helps you to get the breath into your stomach rather than it being stuck in your upper chest. If you watch how people breathe, you'll see that most breathe into their upper chest. However, the bulk of the alveoli sit in the bottom two-thirds of the lungs. These sacks are what exchange the gases needed for many processes in your body. Try to engage them while doing these exercises. Pull the air in deep, try to use the entirety of your lungs. Feel your belly expand as your diaphragm drops down to allow the inhalation. Having your hands on your stomach will help you understand how well you're doing this. And again, don't strain, don't force, don't stress your body out, just play with it and get a good breath in and out.

Preliminary practice for the push breath:

1. Practice this every morning for two weeks and keep notes on how you feel. How does it make you feel? Does it make you feel a little better and more awake in the morning? Does it make you sleepy?
2. Try it before coffee or any caffeine and see if it gives you some pep first.

SEVENTEEN

REWRITING YOUR HISTORY

I WANT TO DISCUSS ONE really interesting series of effects from these methods: you can rewrite your experience of your past. This can be done without going back and remembering it and going over the details. Most people try to get a hold of what happened in the past to try to change it by remembering it over and over and thinking it through. I think of that as the animal part of you rerunning it in your attention to try to feel safer by never letting it go.

If once a wolf came through one particular hole in the fence, then another wolf could at any time. As long as we keep remembering something, we think somehow that will keep that hole closed. Of course, that doesn't work. You just fry your current moment and experience emotional pain, reviewing over and over what happened in the past.

There is some value in that experience, of course. If you review it and find what you missed and then codify the lessons into a new working program for how you are going to function going into the future, it can be of service to you. But then, at that point, you have to be able to set the memory aside and live in the present moment. In some way, that is the trick. How do you set the memory aside? How do you drop it? How can you make it *feel* resolved? In our culture, we tend to look down on feelings and emotions, but they are extremely powerful. If you can honestly feel that your experience in the past is final, the animal and lizard parts of you will get the message. If you only do it intellectually, they can't pick it up. Imagine telling your dog intellectually about something in the past. They won't understand you.

One of the things that needs to happen is that your animal nature has to be able to trust that your higher aspects have things under control. That is something an analysis of the experience—with or without a therapist—can help. Learning how to defend yourself can be of great significance as well. When you really believe you are better prepared, it can help the lizard and animal parts of you to calm down and peacefully do their daily work without needing to be hypervigilant.

By the way, I'd like to briefly explain the difference between the lizard aspects of you and the animal aspects, as I am using it here. The lizard aspects are more about survival, eating, blind reproduction, and base shelter. That's all. It's a one-track mind and a very, very limited consciousness. The animal portion goes beyond the lizard portion similar to the difference between how a snake functions and how wolves or bears function. This portion, of course, still cares about the survival aspects mentioned above but is more aware of social dynamics. It's more worried about hierarchy and position but is also concerned with caring for other pack members. There is somewhat more consideration given to with whom to reproduce. Another interesting way to look at this is in combat—the fighting style of a pack of wolves as compared to that of a cobra. So, animal is more advanced than reptile, but animal consciousness is still rather limited; it cannot project toward the future like human consciousness can. Animals aren't replaying the past and writing down potential solutions for the future.

As a human, you have a very sophisticated nervous system. You have lower aspects and many higher ones. You need them all. Let me repeat: you need them all and you need them all working well together.

There have been moments in my life when the lizard aspects of me alone kept me alive—same thing for my animal aspects. But living in those aspects has some severe downsides as well. You want them available when you need them, but you want them sleeping peacefully by the fire in the corner most of the time. These aspects of you control a great deal of your energy, passion, emotions, and vitality. They are very important in your daily life, but they need to have a specific place in your conscious life, so they don't take over the rest of you. They need to know and understand their place. Better said, *you* need to know and train these parts of you to know their place in how you function.

If they think (it's actually you thinking this) that the higher aspects aren't leading and doing their job correctly, they will take over. This is to help keep you alive, but it will also keep you from thriving and having a satisfying human experience and maybe even a "beyond human experience." There is a wise way in which to live where all these aspects of you live together in the best way possible. This helps all the different aspects of you to do well, which will ultimately give you the best life and best inner-life experience possible. But when they aren't working together, they will create hell inside you, and you will have a rough and painful life. When they aren't working well together you can easily end up anxious, worried, jealous, envious, angry, furious, stuck in the past, terrified of the future, desperately trying to control everyone around you, traumatized, and unable to build a satisfying life.

These concepts of the lizard aspect and the animal aspect are not mine. I learned them from several martial arts teachers as well as a yoga teacher years and years ago. They were part of the traditional teachings, and they hold up well when analyzing the brain. It's a terrible idea to deny any part of you but it's also bad to allow your lizard and animal nature to run your life. You, your consciousness—the most essential part of you—needs to ultimately be running the show, keeping a great household of all these different pieces of you working together in their proper place, keeping them happy and well fed. Do that and you'll have the best chance to have a wonderful inner and outer life.

This brings me back to these methods and rewriting your history. The way you view things, the way you remember things, and the way you imagine things in the future will always be stained by the emotions you feel now as well as what your nervous system is doing now. If you are worried right now and you try to imagine the future, that future will be stained with the emotion of worry and everything you foresee will look bleak. If you remember the past now, you'll get the emotion from back then plus what your nervous system is doing now and what your emotions are doing now. It's an interesting mix of emotions and time. This equation of time plus your emotions is valuable to consider when you're trying to help yourself feel better.

One of the things that really shocked me in my work with these methods is how much they changed what my nervous system is doing now and how much that changed how I see what happened in the past. The past looks different, yet I didn't change or reframe my memories. All of it seems to be rewritten because my nervous system is functioning differently now.

This allows my future to seem far more exciting and satisfying to look toward than it did 10 years ago. Changing how your nervous system works and the brain state you are in matters in every aspect of your life including your past and your future.

This work also seems to have a profound impact on the lizard and animal within me. They seem to be able to relax and chill out and love me the same way a happy dog or cat would. My past had some significant trauma and so my inner life wasn't always like that; in fact, often it was the opposite. So this change has been massive for me and I think it might be massive for many of you too.

Imagine if you could do some work for a while and then look back and see that your history had changed, had somehow been rewritten in a more subjective but not quite delusional way. You're not pretending that things didn't happen, it's just that those memories are colored differently than they used to be. They're no longer all shades of gray and black with danger lurking everywhere, but instead have color and texture and depth and dimension.

You might realize your future begins to seem different to you because you aren't dragging an ugly past around inside and then projecting it and creating it yourself as your future. This change is massive but also shows up somewhat suddenly. It changes your overall experience of life in the most amazing way.

Rewriting and rewiring your past changes everything now and into the future. This method offers an interesting way to change how you function now and the tone of your nervous system, which has a way of recoloring and reordering the past, present, and future.

Questions:

1. Do you think it would be useful in your daily life if you could pull the emotionality out of the past that seems to keep you anchored there?
2. Can you think of a memory that seems to pull at your attention and keeps pulling you into the past? An emotional habit question: does it feel like it almost happens to you?
3. Does it feel like your brain or even your body pulls you to it?

EIGHTEEN

SET TWO OF THE ACTIVATING METHODS

ALL RIGHT, NOW THAT YOU'VE had some time to practice the steps of the Activating Method, let's go a little deeper. We'll go further into the brain itself for our next set of steps. Let me briefly describe a bit about brain anatomy as well as a little bit about the function of the structures that we are going to aim at next.

The occipital lobe[11] is the smallest of the four lobes. It is posterior to the parietal and temporal lobes, and within the skull it lies underneath the occipital bone. The occipital lobe is primarily responsible for visual processing. Occipital lobe lesions can cause visual hallucinations, color agnosia, or agraphia.

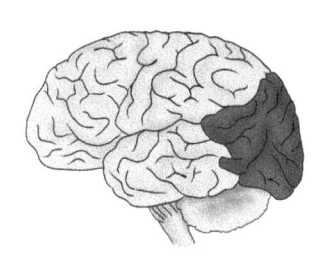

Occipital lobe

The parietal lobe[12] is one of the four major lobes. The parietal lobe is positioned above the temporal lobe and behind the frontal lobe. The major sensory inputs from the skin are received here. The parietal lobe integrates sensory information including spatial sense and navigation. Several areas of the parietal lobe are important in language processing.

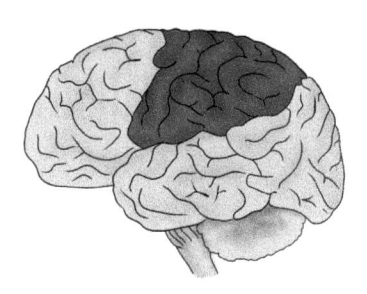

Parietal lobe

The temporal lobe[13] of the brain is sometimes referred to as the neocortex. It forms the cerebral cortex along with the occipital lobe, the frontal lobe, and the parietal lobe. It is anterior to the occipital lobe and posterior to the frontal lobe. The functions of this lobe include speech perception and production, hearing, memory, and some social aspects.

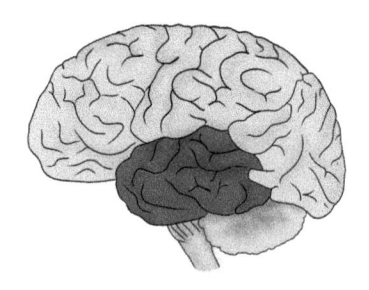

Temporal lobe

The frontal lobe[14] is the largest lobe of the brain, occupying about one-third of the cerebral hemisphere. These paired lobes of the brain lie immediately behind the forehead and include areas concerned with behavior, learning, personality, and voluntary movement. The frontal lobe is the part of the brain that controls important cognitive skills in humans, including emotional expression, some problem solving, memory, judgment, and sexual behaviors.

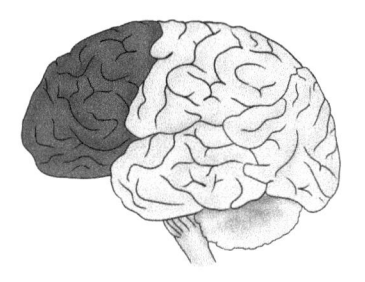

Frontal lobe

In our series of Activating Methods, we are going to move into more areas of the brain. We will be endeavoring to get attention to specific large brain sections to create a little effect. So, we will start working from back to front. The occipital lobe is the farthest back, so let's start there.

1. Sit somewhere comfortable with your spine erect and your attention on the top of your head. Feel suspended from the ceiling.

2. Move your attention from the top of your head to the part of your brain that is just inside the back of your skull and above the spine. Try to get your attention about an inch inside the skull. Remember, you don't need to be perfect, and you aren't trying to become an anatomist. Feel your way to it. Your nervous system knows. I can't stress this point enough. You will tend to want to intellectualize this, and that will keep you from feeling it inside.

3. Hold your attention there for up to a minute. Sometimes it helps to allow some deep breathing to slow your system.

4. Check in on how you feel. Not only are we trying to reconnect with methods to activate our nervous system, but we are also working on finding our way back to being able to feel. This ability to feel has been actively trained out of us in our education. Some of that is good for you and some of it is bad. This is a good way to start practicing taking back your power.

Now that we have worked on the back and lower portions of the brain, let's move to the parietal lobes in the upper and top portions of the brain. (Move forward and up a bit from the occipital lobe.) The parietal lobes are bisected by the corpus callosum, which runs along their length, creating a right and a left hemisphere.

One of my theories with this work is that activating certain aspects of your body—in this case the brain—helps information travel from side to side more easily through repetition and stimulation. That helps signals to move easily through the brain—and the corpus callosum specifically—by getting your attention on both sides simultaneously. Later, I have some interesting physical exercises for helping this connection as well.

For now, if you want to work on this, try executing some of the normal daily actions that you would do with your dominant hand using your non-dominant hand instead. This specific little practice was very helpful for me while I was going through my treatments. It helped my mind clear somewhat during terrible brain fog. It also seemed to help my memory.

1. Sit somewhere comfortable. Lift your head toward the ceiling. Feel suspended and relaxed.
2. Move your attention from the top of your head to the parietal lobes, which sit right under the top of your skull.
3. Gently hold your attention in the lobes for up to a minute—or maybe two if it feels magnetic.
4. Let go of holding your attention and take a few breaths. Check in and

see how you feel. How did activating this area of your body change your experience of yourself and of life?

Going further into the brain, we will next move on to the temporal lobes. If you know where your temples are, you'll be close to the area that we want to work. Your temporal lobes begin behind your temples and then run behind your ears until they meet your occipital lobe in the back. It's a larger area than you might think.

1. Find a comfortable place to sit. Lift the top of your head toward the ceiling. Feel that you're suspended from the top of your head.
2. Draw your attention down from the spot on the top of your head and move it to the part of your brain that is between your temples. Again, let your body and subconscious teach you the right location. You'll know by feel.
3. Hold your attention in this area for up to a minute, longer if it feels important in this area.
4. Allow your hold on your attention to relax and diffuse. Now check in and see how you feel. Checking on how you feel helps you to get a sense, over time, for what these methods are doing for you and what areas have specific effects for you.
5. Remember to be playful with these exercises and not make them "hard work."

From there we will go to the last position in this row of Activating Methods. We are going to focus on the most forward part of the brain, conveniently known as the frontal lobe. This lobe houses the most evolved parts of your brain so it's important to be sure to activate this area. It basically sits right behind your forehead, which is one of the reasons why traumatic head injury can cause such an interesting change in personality. It can be stunning to see the change in people you've known for years after a significant enough force applied to this part of the brain. They may never be the same again.

1. Hopefully you are catching the theme by now. These methods are best learned when sitting in a quiet place, back erect and upright. Roll the hips gently forward to help straighten the back and to allow certain things to happen at the tailbone area, specifically at the sacrum.
2. Feel like the top of your head is suspended from the ceiling—just a nice, pleasant, uplifting feeling.
3. Move your attention to the space right behind your frontal bone, your forehead. Go inside, an inch or two behind the bone. Don't worry about being super specific.
4. Coax your attention to stay in this area for up to a minute or longer until you feel satisfied it's done. If you don't feel satisfied after more than two minutes, move on anyway, at least at this stage of learning. More is not always better. Sometimes it actively messes things up and destroys what you are trying to accomplish. This is not stuff to push and mess around with—take your time and allow it to open up to you. Don't force it.
5. Relax and take a few nice breaths and again take a moment to notice how your body and your emotions feel. Observe what your mind is doing and what thoughts are going through it. You might even find that there are no thoughts at all, which is a wonderful thing if that happens.

This is a good place to stop these methods to practice what you've learned and see how they work for you. The Activating Methods are fairly comprehensive and take some time to learn properly. It also takes daily practice to be able to do them well and without much thought. So, take some time to practice these and the others you've learned, and we will build on these foundations that we are laying now.

I made this method to be as complete and powerful as I possibly could, and ultimately I'm not holding any of it back. I am trying to pass it on to you intelligently and wisely so that you can learn it and get the most out of it.

Please be sure to practice what you've learned and be careful not to take too big a bite all at once. Activating has to be practiced enough and understood well enough that it becomes alive within you. It won't work as a theory, and it won't work as memorized knowledge. This has to become part of you and a living part of your experience.

For daily practice at this point:

1. Do the first row of the Activating Methods in the morning.
2. Do the second row in the evening. Practice them separately for a while to see how they affect you. Later, I'll show you how to put them together.

Start now and try to find a way to practice them every day until they become a habit. The results from these come over time and through practice, so be patient; you are ultimately rewiring parts of your nervous system. For me, going to bed at night and waking up in bed in the morning are regular habits that remind me to practice. But do whatever works for you.

NINETEEN

"MIND STORM," MEMORY, AND ANXIETY

MIND FOG IS A FAIRLY common phrase you might often hear in the health industry. But mind fog is a terribly inadequate phrase for what is actually a whole category of mental and energy problems. It is certainly true that there is something like a fog that blocks your ability to think and so everything is a little nondescript, hard to see, hidden, obscured, and hard to get your mind around. And maybe that's all it is for many people. But for me, there was way more going on in a similar vein and that seems to me to be connected. For me, it was definitely also painful physically, mentally, and emotionally. It's not just about being "foggy" and somewhat unperceptive; there's a lot more going on.

Perhaps "mind storm" is a better term. You can't see through it, it comes at you and disturbs your peace, it can be quite painful like lightning striking the ground or hail pounding on your house. For some people it *is* like fog, passively blocking them. But for some I believe the term mind storm is much more accurate and might help others realize what is going on with them.

I think many people divorce the pain of a mind storm from the inability to perceive and just call the pain a headache or migraine or even something like fibromyalgia because it isn't entirely located in the head. I can understand that it's helpful to break things down to treat them more specifically. But I do believe the fog can be connected to the pain rather than the two being separate phenomena. Although it doesn't sound terribly unpleasant, mind fog can be deeply, deeply painful. You can't do normal everyday things, it takes the computer that is your mind and denies access to it, it brutalizes your sense of self and self-worth, and you begin to lose yourself, which is a particular kind of hell.

It also deeply affects your memory. That is in part because when your mind is foggy you produce, at best, foggy new memories. But it messes with your recovery and perception of old memories as well. It's a fairly unpleasant experience to live through. Memories provide a context for everything else in your life. Without some of that knowledge, you are always starting over again, at least on some level. When you can't think clearly, you miss context as well as the capacity to think your way through and around things. That combination of factors brings a level of high anxiety and, at least on occasion, a fair amount of anger as you realize what is going on with you.

Anxiety, fear, and anger don't feel good. They wear you down and, over time, they damage your body. It's very difficult to feel a sense of peace, the way you treat yourself and others changes for the worse, and you move further and further away from who you really are.

Partly, I wanted to go into some detail here because some readers might know someone who is going through something like this, and this will help them understand a bit about what's happening. It's a bigger problem than you might imagine. I hope none of you reading this will ever have to experience it.

Fortunately, there are ways out of it. Depending on what is causing these experiences, there are several things that can help. Please talk to your doctor, and if the first one can't help you, look for another. There are many things you can do to help yourself as well. Sleep matters a lot as does true, peaceful rest. Good diet, focusing on the nutrients you need, is also very important. Supplements can be very helpful. Getting out of stressful environments and relationships can also be crucial. My system in general has been a huge benefit for me in this regard and the methods in this book pulled me back into the light. So, there is hope. Don't lose hope.

There is an important detail that I'd like to mention here because when people talk about "positive emotions," some people will translate this in their minds as useless, not important, ineffective advice. But that simply is not true. Your emotions matter. The way you feel has a huge effect on your life. It will change your capacities. It will change how your mind works. It will change how your memory works. It will dictate huge parts of all your relationships, especially with yourself.

If you want to heal, it is absolutely crucial that you start to focus on building positive emotional states in yourself. Happiness, satisfaction, love, belief, faith, care, peace, calm, bliss, even ecstasy are states that you want to start to court in your experience. Remember, don't try to force them. You have to court them and do the right things to bring them into your experience.

For a long time, people have been convinced—and in many ways taught—that emotions don't matter, are completely uncontrollable, and that they don't change your overall experience of life. But I think this deeply disempowers you. This gives others more control over you. This makes you much less than you could be. Yet people keep programming everyone's mental software to believe that emotions don't matter.

Most people who say that don't even think about it. It just comes out because they've been saying it for so long. They haven't spent any real time exploring for themselves if it is in fact true. They aren't the ones trying to disempower you. They are already disempowered and are passing that computer software in their mind along like a computer virus.

Your emotions are one of the most powerful things about you, but you do need to get in touch with them, understand them, define what you're feeling so that you can conduct them wisely. I talk about this in more detail in my book *Ah, Brain, Why Do You Trouble Me So Much?* And later, in more books, courses, and videos I will talk about emotions in detail, so stay tuned if you're interested. For now, realize your emotions matter a great deal, especially when trying to conquer the mind storm, memory problems, and free-floating anxiety.

There is hope. Begin to believe in that.

I added these chapters about health in this book because I want to give people hope. I also want to convey my conviction that these methods might also help keep people from having all the kinds of health problems that show up. There are preventative practices that might be useful across the board for people long term.

1. Do you believe that you can feel better through your own efforts?
2. If you don't believe that you could feel better, regardless of whether you are starting off in great health or in bad health, what do you think you are telling your brain and nervous system to do? (We might call this psychosomatic in a dismissive way, but maybe it is worth taking some time to consider whether this has an impact on you.)
3. Do you think your brain has an impact on the rest of you and on your life? Do you believe your thoughts are in any way affecting your brain?

TWENTY

FOR A BETTER LIFE

ULTIMATELY, ALL THE WORK WE are doing in this book is to help you have a better life. All the exercises are aimed at giving you better control over your inner environment. Many of us have gotten stuck in certain repetitive loops within our nervous system, brain states, neurochemistry, and hormones. A lot of this habitual and repetitive looping in how our system works is due to stress. It's due to watching how other people in our life function and copying them. It's due to our acting in automatic and unconscious ways.

It's actually fairly interesting for me at this point in my life, having worked on these methods for most of my lifetime, to see how much modern society trains us away from observing and working consciously with our inner environment. It's somewhat unbelievable to me that when I say "inner environment" people don't know what I mean. They don't realize how powerful and large their mind is. They don't see how incredibly sophisticated and informative their emotions are. They don't realize all the amazing things that are working within their body. They don't see how much their life will change by working within themselves and inside their bodies as I am trying to elucidate in this book. These changes can radically change your life, how you function, how you feel, and your ultimate capacity as a human being.

All of modern life seems to be directed toward keeping your attention outside of yourself.

Of course, if I think about this it's somewhat easy to understand why. If people can keep your attention outside of you, they can direct you in certain ways. For example, they can get you to buy things through product placement. They can get you to vote for certain things through creating massive fear in the news. They can get you to work for them even in ways that don't serve you.

This is actually the most fundamental sort of resource that a human has: Is your attention being directed by you or is it being directed by others?

Your life goes where you put your attention, or where your attention gets drawn. Your mind is like a creation machine. It will create with whatever information, images, sounds, and smells you give it. You give things to your mind through your attention, whether that attention is outside of the objective world or inside your thoughts, imagination, emotions, feelings, energies, and sensations.

Large parts of your mind don't know the difference between something experienced outside of you or inside of you. That means you have abilities to change yourself and your life through what you produce and experience inside.

You could consider this mental or emotional practice. For example, when I was getting ready to audition for college entrance exams on the piano, my piano teacher suggested that I spend time away from the piano and play the songs in my mind: to actually see my hands play through the songs, see the sheet music in my mind, and so on. This practice made me a much better pianist than I was previously. In fact, it seemed my skill level got significantly better from this practice at that point in my development. I realized later that if I added strong emotional content to this practice, I got significantly better results.

The combination of consciously working with your mind and emotions together is massively powerful, but, interestingly, almost no one does this. The yoga masters talk about it, martial arts masters talk about it, musical masters talk about it, artists talk about it, athletes talk about it, but outside of chasing these endeavors at the highest levels, the average person doesn't really know about it.

In fact, it seems to me they are actively trained away from it. "Your emotions don't matter," "your feelings don't matter," "stop ignoring everyone and thinking you have better things to do," (and usually the things to do are things they want from you that serve them and rarely you).

Can you get lost in your mind and get nothing accomplished in your life? Absolutely. But to ignore this powerful aspect of who and what you are is one of the most—if not *the* most—disempowering things that can happen to you as a human being. If you can turn the tide and direction of your mind and emotions and energies inside, it will absolutely and without fail change how you function in life.

This is the crux of self-improvement and changing your life for the better. If you don't change the programs in your mind and habits of your emotions and the use of whatever energy you have in your life, you will never be any different and you'll always have the same results as you had before. If you take lots of action without first changing the programming, you will create

whatever you were creating faster and on a bigger scale. If you have the right programming, that will be wonderful. However, if you have the wrong programming, you will build destruction, pain, and suffering for those around you faster and more powerfully. Action matters a lot but the underlying programming matters more.

Imagine if you will, a supercomputer faster than any other computer on Earth and more powerful than any three put together. What that computer can do will still be 100% determined by the programs that run it. If you put useful programming in it, you'll get superfast and super powerful desired results from the supercomputer. If you put damaging programming in it—let's say programming that will damage all the electrical grids on the planet—it will destroy power grids faster, more powerfully, and, in a way, more creatively than any other.

In that case, a slower, less powerful computer will in fact be a benefit because it won't enact the poor programming as fast or as powerfully. We always think of intelligence as being this wonderful thing, but with poor mental and emotional programming, poor attention, and poor conclusions drawn from data, a superfast mind will create destruction and damage much, much faster than a slower mind. All power can be used in some positive way, or it can be used for destruction and mayhem. You can build a bookshelf with a power saw, but you can also cut your fingers off.

What is going on in your mind, what is going on in your emotions, and what is going on with your energies—however you view the potential energy your system has to use—is extraordinarily important for your life. It's extraordinarily important inside of you—in your mind and emotions—and outside of you—in your house, your work, your family, and your environment.

But for some reason we don't really see this. We don't see the importance of changing that inner programming and our habitual ways of using our emotions and energies. And if you try to get it across to people, they say it's not practical or it's just New Age crap or psychology mumbo-jumbo or time wasting.

Why are we all so reticent to make our inner life a priority?

Why don't we take advantage of working with the aspects of ourselves that could make a huge difference in the experience of our lives?

Why do we wildly disempower ourselves?

Ultimately, the Nytality Method is my attempt to solve this for myself and my attempt to truly help others solve this problem. It's worked absolutely brilliantly—although at times slowly—as I figured it out in the lab that is myself and my life. I hope it will work for others too.

Your inner life not only matters; it's your access point to how you create every aspect of your life that is in your control.

Questions for leading a better life:

1. What could you change today that would help you get better control of your life's questions?
2. What distractions could you eliminate today that would allow you to work with your own emotions and mind?

TWENTY-ONE

THE MENINGES MEDITATION

WITHIN YOUR SPINE YOU HAVE three layers of tissue that help to protect your spinal cord and that contain cerebrospinal fluid.[15] Collectively we call these the meninges.[16] These layers also cover your brain inside your skull. Meningitis is an infection in this area of the body. It is excruciating and can be deadly.

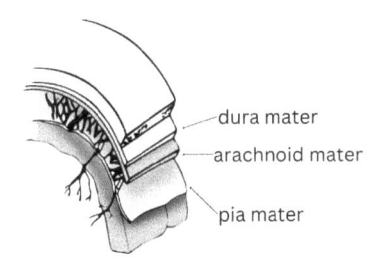

Meninges

The outermost layer is called the dura mater, the middle layer is called the arachnoid mater, and the innermost layer is called the pia mater.[17] We are going to use these three layers of tissue within the spine to build a profound meditation process that has proven to be very valuable to me in changing my brain states, in helping me reach stillness, and in helping my body and my brain heal.

This meditation isn't hard to do or understand, but being patient enough to work the process can be a little tough for people looking for instant results. With continued practice over the course of time—like most other things in this method and in life—the benefits will blossom within and around you. Many people don't like this sort of flowery language, perhaps because the parts of their brains that appreciate beauty, color, and artistry have become dormant either due to neglect and poor education, or because life has traumatized and beat them into a deep emergency mode. I am trying to help you wake that part of your brain up. It is very important and makes life more beautiful for you.

Many men have been taught that artistic, flowery, soft activities are somehow unmanly as well, but it is interesting that at some point in many incredible martial arts they require you to become engaged in some form of art like poetry, flower arranging, or music. Let me needle the tough people (all people because it's definitely not just a male thing) a bit: it's a bit wimpy to not be willing to engage all of you, including those pesky emotions. By the way, I'm not mocking you, it's just that sometimes the only way to reach someone who is shutting large chunks of themselves off is to push them in their "toughness."

Truth be told, you are missing important aspects of yourself if you are unwilling to handle your emotions wisely or work to understand all the dimensions of life and most especially of you. Sometimes, personal development and meditation get lumped into the category of airy-fairy useless nonsense. But I can't think of anything more difficult than learning to rule yourself and becoming a monarch in your own inner kingdom or queendom or whatever medieval term you want to use.

THE MENINGES MEDITATION

Rule is probably the wrong term. What you actually want to do is something more like orchestrate or conduct. What you think of as yourself isn't all of you. You can't just force yourself to do or be or emote willy-nilly. Those things require a lot more coaxing, rewarding, building, and encouraging than "rule" would suggest. The force mechanism isn't enough—you need to plant, nurture, and grow seeds. People tend to worship force and miss the importance of planting seeds and nurturing growth. Chasing instant results can destroy you. Learning to grow things, learning to attract things, learning to cultivate and develop can change your entire life.

On to the meditation:

1. Sit up straight just as you have in the other methods.
2. On your next inhale, run your breath from your tailbone up around your skull on the inside of the bone. Get used to the inhale moving up your spine.
3. On the exhale, run your breath from around your brain under the skull bones down the inside of the spine to your tailbone.
4. Inhale up and exhale down. Practice a few rounds of this until you get the hang of it.
5. Once you get the hang of it, put your attention on the dura mater and run your breath along this tissue from your tailbone to around your brain in the skull.
6. Run your breath along the same tissue from your brain down your spine to the tailbone.
7. Move on to the arachnoid mater, the middle layer of the meninges.
8. Run your breath up the middle layer on the in breath and down the middle layer on the out breath.
9. Move down to the deepest layer of the meninges, the pia mater.
10. Run your breath up the deepest layer on the in breath and down the

deepest layer on the out breath.

11. When you finish this, go back to the outside layer and start the process again, outside to inside.
12. Repeat this cycle for a while until you feel like you got something done. This can be a few minutes to hours depending on how you feel and your current goals.

Remember, this isn't about perfection in your understanding of anatomy. It's about creating a feeling in your system and using that to have an impact on your inner world. These layers of tissue are actually very close together, but we are using our mind and our anatomy to create a cool effect and begin the process of being absorbed into meditation.

This specific meditation was very important for me in healing the problems I had with Lyme disease as well as a number of other infections. If you are someone who has had chronic health problems, this might be amazingly helpful in your recovery. It certainly was profound for me in that way. Please take this slowly. It is powerful in some interesting ways.

This meditation was also very profound for me in terms of the creation of altered states (sometimes known as mystical states or spiritual states). Experiencing these will change your life in ways that I can't even begin to describe. I hope you will undertake the journey for

yourself. The impact you can make on yourself in just this meditation is deeply profound, but when you put it together with the other methods, you can truly change everything about how you experience yourself and life.

I hope you will get a lot out of this.

How to practice the Meninges Meditation:

Take a few minutes in the afternoon today and practice this meditation.

How do you feel afterward?

Try to do this every day for a few weeks, ideally at the same time each day. This will help you see what results it gives you. You want to train your body and specifically your nervous system to employ this technique in your life. If you do it regularly and (more powerfully) at the same time each day, it will almost happen by itself. It's a cool feeling to have it take off on its own.

TWENTY-TWO

THE EMPOWERED BREATH METHOD

THIS BREATHING METHOD IS SOMEWHERE between breath work, meditation, and pranayama. Its impact is deep and quite powerful, so I hope you will take it with enough weight to focus on doing it properly without being "serious" about it and straining. It had a wildly strong impact on me when I finally put it together in this form.

You'll notice with all the breathing methods included in this book that none of them control the timing of the inhalation and exhalation or the hold out or in. And this is a very important thing to point out. Breathing methods are quite powerful, they work at the intersection of what is voluntary and involuntary within you, so they have a large impact on your nervous system as well as the acidity in your system.

In order to do methods that control the timing of the different aspects of the breath, you would need to know what state your nervous system is in. And you would need to know how alkaline or acidic your system is and if that acidity/alkalinity is being driven by changes in the oxygen and carbon dioxide exchange. You would need to know how your nervous system is tuned, as in sympathetically dominant or maybe overly lax. You would also need to account for the effect of diet changes on your chemistry, sleep patterns, and the states of your overall energy system.

All these aspects were noted to be very important when they were imparted to me by a few of my teachers. So, this is more complicated than most people recognize, and once you realize where you are in relation to these factors, you need to know which parts of the breathing pattern to change in order to attain the changes you want. It's a rather complicated area of science. I wanted to point this out because human beings aren't all the same. In fact, we have lots of things going on within us. Authenticity to who and what we are in our system and how it functions are important.

So, I have not included any such timed-breath methods in this book. All these breath methods should be done at your pace and to the pace your body, nervous system, and subconscious dictate. Please don't force or try to control your breathing at the expense of your health and personal development. You can throw yourself off if you try to force and control the breath. Let the breath show you. Let the breath work open you up to your higher self and let that direct you. The highest part of you knows what you need, you simply need to listen for it.

For this we will start the same way that we do most of the other methods as we learn them.

1. Find somewhere comfortable to sit, roll your hips forward, make your spine straight without force or tension. Feel like your head is suspended from the ceiling.
2. Take an in breath and "feel" the air go up your spine.
3. Contract the bottom of your pelvis in the space between your genitals and your anus, the perineum. This is a very light contraction, just enough to say you did it and no more than that. You're actually getting some nice movement in some important muscles like levator ani and pubococcygeus. Our ultimate intent, however, is to make some

changes in the nervous system as we move up the spine to nerve and hormonal centers. We are also moving energy up the spine to the brain, if that makes sense to you.

4. During the same breath and after step 3, try to contract the space on the front of your sacrum and the front side of the back of your pelvis as well as the front side of the vertebrae in your lower back, the lumbar spine. There is an interesting muscle group here consisting of the iliacus and the psoas muscles, which together are called the iliopsoas. Again, this is just a light contraction. Now, you can go crazy trying to isolate these muscles if you get carried away. Make it simple so you can feel it and just try to do it. Your body already knows, it's just your intellect that doesn't. Allow your body to teach your consciousness. Try to create a light contraction on the front of the tailbone, front side of the back of your pelvis, as well as the front side of the spine in your lower back. It's much much easier to do that than to describe in words. Play with it.

5. Now, after step 4, still on the in breath, contract the area of your solar plexus toward your spine and try to get some of that contraction on the front side of the spine opposite the solar plexus. This will stimulate the pancreas (a part of the endocrine system that has to do with hormones) as well as the celiac nerve plexus. It also has a wonderful toning effect on the vagus nerve.

6. After step 5, on the same breath, we want to feel a little contraction on the upper third of the chest bone (sternum) right above the thymus, as well as a contraction on the front of the spine directly opposite and a little bit above the thymus near the C7, T1, and T2 vertebrae. This will stimulate all kinds of cool structures within your nervous system and hormonal system. (Remember all I'm saying here is that we are working on stimulating the structure with our attention and contraction.) Again, this is a light contraction, just enough to say it happened.

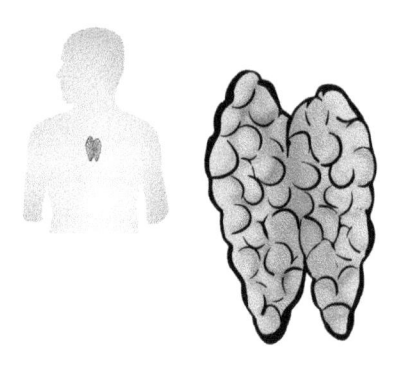

Thymus

7. After step 6 we go on to the throat. Here we want to create a light contraction right at the midpoint and center of the throat, as well as a very, very light contraction on the upper two vertebrae and lowest part of the back of the skull. This will cover the thyroid and the junction of your spine and skull. Be very, very easy with this. The contraction is like closing your eyelid, not like holding onto something with your hand.

8. This will bring our breath up to the brain and the top of the head. We want to hold our breath for just a comfortable amount of time when our attention reaches this area. Just enjoy the feeling of having lifted the breath and energy up to your brain and the top area of your head.

9. Exhale easily and without rushing. Start the same sequence with the next inhale.

As you learn these, feel free to practice one individually and practice another one as you work through the breath and figuring out how to hold a little tension in the area described. Play with it for a while and be careful not to overdo it. There's a lot going on with this kind of work and hopefully you will find out for yourself by taking the information and steps described and practicing them wisely until you get a result.

None of this is rocket science and it's actually much harder to describe than to do. After a while, this method happens by itself when you sit down to do it. Once you get good at it, you can do it anywhere and in many positions, although your spine does need to be straight and you do need to be relaxed.

There have been methods similar to this going back thousands of years in India, China, the Middle East, and in many other places. There is a good reason for this as they have a profound impact. There are many people in the modern world who are discovering this more through the lens of science than, say, the traditions of yesteryear, but however you get to this, the results come from the *doing*, not from the *knowing*.

You can do as many repetitions as you like once you get good at it, but give yourself some time so you do not force it and strain your system as you make changes. I would start with three repetitions a day for a week or two. Then you could move up to nine a day and run that for several months. After that, do what feels right to you. Never do more than what feels right to you at any moment. If it feels like the wrong time or you're doing too many, stop. Let your system guide you.

Many of you will probably want to take this to the extreme. Sometimes I do too and there is a time for this but please be careful—this is powerful, I would dare to say wildly powerful. Take your time, don't rush it, and don't force it. The right amount is always massively better than overdoing. Overdoing it can kill your results as well as potentially hurt you. I don't believe these to be in any way inherently dangerous, but I do think it's worth a warning.

In my experience, methods like this tend to exaggerate who you are inside, so please be sure to take good care of yourself inside. That way, you don't become a problem to others on the outside when you supercharge yourself with these kinds of methods.

In a few traditions I've studied, the teachers are very explicit and tell their students that these methods will take what you are inside and make you much more of it. I've definitely seen this happen within some ancient traditions. In fact, that's often why some of those methods are almost never taught. One of my yoga teachers had seven students before me and all of them failed to get past the first level. He said they couldn't handle the power it gave them. Basically, they became arrogant jerks. I met them at a party once and I would have to concur with that assessment. They were clearly arrogant.

However, the methods I'm presenting here work more slowly and in a more stable way. I very much prefer this to the other method I mentioned above, which was like drinking jet fuel. You'd better have your system functioning well or it could become a problem for you. My way is to fix the holes in your health, fix the holes in your inner world, and then add more jet fuel once you have a handle on yourself. It's another approach that a teacher of mine talked about in their teaching.

This method is powerful but also quite safe and measured. It is based on anatomical understanding and what happens when you use your physical, mental, emotional, and energetic resources to create a flowering of the potential of your system. It's truly beautiful to see the changes it can create within you.

How to practice:

This method is best practiced when things are quiet and you won't be distracted. Try to wake up a few minutes early tomorrow. Then work through the empowered breath technique a few times —or, if you're up for it, try to run through it nine times. If you can work through it before you do anything else in your day, it is a little easier to feel what it does to your nervous system.

TWENTY-THREE

WHY IS THIS BOOK DIFFERENT FROM THE FIRST TWO?

IN MY FIRST TWO BOOKS, I started teaching my work with one specific system of principles applied in two different ways. In the first book, I applied them to dieting, and in the second book, to debugging your mental and emotional software in a general way. I had an original plan for how I wanted to release the information in my system, but as the system grew and developed, I began to see a different path that would lead to more efficient and stable progress for the greatest number of people.

I began to see a little more clearly that it would be helpful to work on the "software" and the "hardware" together, rather than focusing in one area and coming back to the other. My perspective also changed as I developed more methods that were easier to teach, especially to people completely unfamiliar with many of the more unusual aspects of my system.

So, for this book, I decided to pivot and change up the way I present the material. I also decided that I would need to teach more in other areas—not just in written word form—sooner than I had originally planned. This would allow me to reach more people quickly, and to reach people who don't like to read or who have set up their life with many distractions that would make reading practically impossible.

One of the things that makes changing your life difficult is that your nervous system can become physically locked into certain habits and ways of functioning. And while deep changes can happen by working with the software, sometimes working with the hardware moves things

faster for some people. The two combine and synergize really well to make radical changes quickly.

Here's how the methods in this book apply to the methods in the first two books: the stress of being locked down in your nervous system and brain states will make dieting harder and will make gaining life perspective very difficult. We are actively trying to reset some aspects of the nervous system processes to relieve how it is locked down.

As your nervous system is able to reset and get out of emergency mode—hypervigilance, free-floating anxiety, bursts of anger and frustration—it will become easier to manage your diet as well as gain a larger life perspective. When you're under a lot of stress, your body begins to look for cheap energy sources like sugar, energy drinks, salty foods, and so on. So, learning how to actively reset your nervous system through your own efforts can be one of the best things to do to change your diet. There's also something to be said for how your body will want to react when it feels like it's always on a battlefield: It will want to hoard resources. In your body that can mean storing fat. This is not the only potential response and adaptation, but it can be a big one. It's worth considering what that means in regard to diet and weight loss as well as the importance of learning to work with your mind and emotions. There's an intimate connection between the two.

It's also hard to think of the big picture when you're on a battlefield or at least feel like you are. It doesn't matter exactly where you are, but, rather, how you feel and think about where you are. Some people can do very well under extremely trying circumstances while others will struggle under the best possible circumstances.

Everyone isn't built the same, they aren't given the same education and training, and the neurochemistry isn't always the same. So, there is no value here in shame, guilt, or blame. You can't start from anywhere but exactly where you are.

The real lesson to learn here is that you can change what's going on *inside* you to have better resilience and the ability to move forward with what's going on *outside* of you. You are far more powerful than you think. You are far more capable than you think. But you will have to change something about how you think, emote, and act if you want something in your life to change.

You have to change something to get different results. Then you have to look at those results and adapt because you might not go exactly where you want on the first try—you might have to play with it for a while. The first step is realizing that *you can change things*. Then take a step—any step—to actively change something in your mind or your emotions or your body. Just start somewhere and then, every day, keep moving forward in some way. Be careful about emotionalizing everything because that is a sure-fire way to make it harder to move forward.

My first two books are built to help you to debug your programming and bring more energy into the system. The work in this book is more about rewiring the hardware in your body and allowing that to change things—that is how it all plays out in my experience.

Imagine refurbishing your computer, giving it more power, a better cooling system, more RAM, more memory, better cables, and a more stable electric supply. Then you go through and take out all the buggy programming and reinstall each system with new updated software. What kind of change would that make to your experience with your computer? That is something we're trying to accomplish in ourselves with this work.

This will change your experience of life dramatically in the same way that changing your computer system and its programming will change your Internet or work experience. The difference can blow your mind. But because it's intangible, it's hard for people to see and measure correctly. People are absolutely obsessed with tangibles even though the intangibles we possess as humans are true wealth or a potential hell, depending on how we use them.

Ultimately you want to refurbish the computer and remove buggy software and install properly working and well-organized software in order to change your life experience. All my methods are designed to work in an integrated fashion to accomplish this in you: mentally, emotionally, physically, and energetically.

If you skip aspects of it and only work on one piece—for example, if you only like the physical methods or the emotional methods—you will leave lots of potential suffering in your experience because all the aspects play a part in your life experience as well as your life success.

But any work will help and will start to change the whole. Start somewhere and begin the journey toward reworking how you function and rediscovering more of who and where you are.

I personally think this is the greatest adventure that a human being can undertake. It also comes with the greatest potential treasure.

Give it a shot. You can do this—yes, you—right where you are, right as you are. You can accomplish something with this right now.

TWENTY-FOUR

OCCUPY ALL OF YOU

OCCUPY ALL THE ROOMS OF the house inside you.

This is a metaphor that I have read in at least three separate texts—one ancient and two written in the last 200 years. This will serve us well here because it isn't always easy to see what is going on within you. It's helpful to engage the nonlinear, more abstract part of your mind through metaphor and imagery.

One way to look at yourself and your functions is to consider yourself a house. Most people believe themselves to be in a studio apartment. They are living in one room and thinking that is the whole of themselves. And because of that, they don't go looking for doors and windows to the other rooms within them. They might not even realize that they have a kitchen or a bathroom, so they don't know how to feed themselves or get rid of the waste and toxins.

Some people see themselves as a house with two rooms and a bathroom and kitchen. They can access more of themselves and their functions. Life is better and more comfortable for them.

Others relate to themselves in the world as if all they are is a body or all they are is a mind or all they are is a bunch of moving passions and emotions. They might hear about the other places—the mind or emotions or whatever parts they don't relate to—but they can't access them. They don't know how to live within themselves, and they don't know how to open the door in a useful way.

Some people know intuitively that their studio has more rooms or that their house has more rooms, and they are desperate to find the doors and the keys or a window to get into them. They ask everyone they know, yet no one else knows how to get from room to room either.

Then they might read something or hear someone describe how to go from room to room. And they might seek out teachers who can teach them how to open the doors, find the keys, turn on the heat, and turn on the lights. Most people probably think they understand all about how they function—or perhaps that's not the right way to say it. It's more like they are not conscious of the possibilities and within themselves they feel like they have some kind of handle on their whole self. And they probably do…in one room.

They might also meet someone who thinks they have themselves and their life all together. Beware of this person because their ego has overrun the unique individual that they actually are. So far as I can tell, this inflated ego is the death of any future growth and the most obvious signs that someone is misusing their inner world.

Earlier, I mentioned a yoga teacher I worked with who said all his previous students became untrainable. This is what happened to all of them; in different ways and on different levels, this was the essence of their deviation in themselves from the training they'd had. I met all of them and it was subtle but startling: I could hear them talking about how special they are and how they should have special "perks" in life. They were so wonderful now, in their view, they didn't need to work on themselves, be of service, or ever have to work to make money again. They believed they'd had all the training from that system, but none of them got past level one. Be careful when you start to believe yourself superior or somehow better than others. You've just shut yourself off from the most wonderful things life has to offer.

But let's get back to the metaphor because there is more to say and understand. It's possible to learn where the rooms are within you, how to turn on the lights, how to cook, how to use the bathroom, how to do your laundry, how to sleep in the bedroom, and how to keep it clean. It's helpful to have a teacher but it's not impossible to do this on your own, because you have guidance within you.

There is a part of you that can teach you all you need to know about where you live and who you are. This part of you is substantially bigger than you might think and includes things like hunches, inclinations, inspiration, intuition, certainty, vision, and just a deep sense of knowing. This master panel to you and your house is within you if you can learn to tune in.

As you develop, you can begin to see not only that you do not live in a studio but that you don't live in a two-room house either. You live in a massive mansion with a huge estate. You discover that you have so many more rooms in your house and so much more land than you can currently believe if you can figure out how to go from room to room or get in touch with the guidance within you to reclaim the familiar and claim the new aspects of you.

Some of these rooms are rather obvious when you hear about them. Knowing how to use them and their location within you allows you to consciously expand your use of them. Some of the rooms you wouldn't believe are even possible to house within a human being—but you won't understand that until you open the door within yourself to experience them.

The Nytality Methods are an attempt to build a floor plan and a staircase to experience more of your house and more of you. It's not the only method—there are several of them out there all over the world and going back into prehistory.

Surprisingly often, people think that they and they alone have the method to "explore your house," but the truth comes from inside. Anyone can source it. It's actually built into who and what we are. There is already the thread of connection. But these methods can help you find your way. And they only matter if you use them to actually walk your way on your path.

Explore, my friend, explore.

How to practice:

Take five minutes sometime today when you can pay attention and see if you can label what emotions you are experiencing. During that five minutes, see if you can also watch your thoughts, maybe even write a few down. And if you really want to test yourself during these five minutes, also try to experience your body. Something really interesting happens when you watch all three aspects of yourself concurrently. This might sound easy to do, but you have been trained not to see what is going on within you. It might take some time to really experience these aspects of yourself, especially all three together.

TWENTY-FIVE

THE FINAL SERIES OF THE ACTIVATING METHODS

NOW WE WILL GO DEEPER into the brain to reach more structures with our work.

The pituitary gland[18]

Your pituitary gland is about the size of a pea and is situated in a bony hollow, just behind the bridge of your nose. It is attached to the base of your brain. The pituitary gland is often called the "master gland" because it controls several other hormone glands, including the thyroid, adrenals, testicles, and ovaries.

Hormones are chemicals that carry messages from one cell to another through your bloodstream.

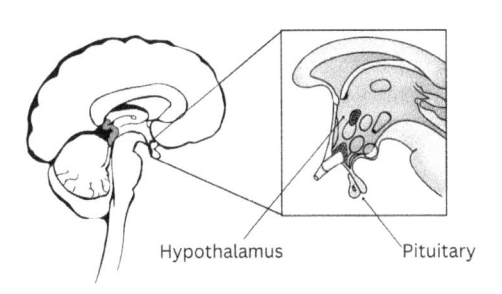

Pituitary & hypothalamus

The hypothalamus[19]

The hypothalamus, which controls the pituitary by sending messages, is situated immediately above the pituitary gland. This serves as a communications center for the pituitary gland, by sending hormonal messages as signals.

The pineal gland[20]

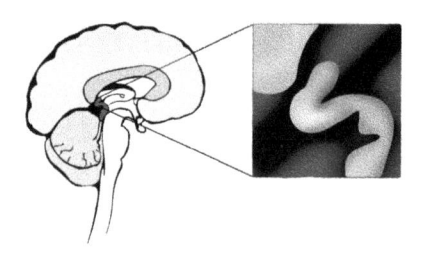

Pineal gland

The pineal gland is a small, pine-cone-shaped organ that lies within the roof of the third ventricle (fluid-filled space) deep within the brain. Studies have shown that, on average, the size of the pineal gland is similar to a grain of rice. It is located within an area called the epithalamus, just behind the thalamus and above the cerebellum, resting at the back of the brain, near the brain stem.

Earlier, we worked through the lobes of the brain. Now we will move on to work through the hormonal centers, or glands, listed above. Gland work can have extraordinary results if you practice it regularly and make it a real part of your life. You'd be surprised how many great things can come from it. We are only at the beginning stage of gland work in this book, but these methods are still very powerful.

People often turn to drugs to improve how they feel and to experience altered states of consciousness. I definitely understand the drive to feel better and expand your consciousness and what you can perceive. It's one of the reasons I put these methods together, because with what is in this book, I can create exceptional and unusual states of consciousness for myself. The change it makes in my daily life is the consciousness version of going from making $30,000 to $300,000 a year. Even someone who has never experienced these states has gotten a taste of such experiences when they were in love, accomplished something great, were in the height of sex, or maybe through the power of music.

The really cool thing about what we're trying to accomplish here is that, with practice, you can create these experiences without the need for anything external. You won't need the love from someone else, the satisfaction of achieving an outside aim, sex, or even music. All those things are wonderful and I'm not in any way telling you not to have those in your life. But what I do want to give you is the possibility to create those states and experiences in yourself through your own efforts inside.

It seems to me a great deal of the odd or even dangerous behavior in humans comes from their desperate attempts to figure out how to change how they feel inside. A great deal of that behavior comes from people trying to control others so that they can feel powerful, or produce serotonin or large adrenaline dumps. How much of that crazy behavior—I'm calling it crazy because it often leads to self-destruction, jail time, terrible accidents, slavery, rape, wars, and even death—could be ameliorated by the ability of people to directly change their states inside?

I suppose I see this as somewhat of a conscious, revolutionary, and evolutionary choice that humans can make. I'm not sure that environmental pressures are enough to create this evolutionary upgrade within humans or, more specifically, for themselves during their lifetime. Perhaps there is a stage where humanity needs to consciously choose to upgrade itself through its own efforts. If you want these benefits, you'll have to choose to make these changes yourself through your own efforts and expanding of consciousness.

This is why I'm not very enthusiastic about making these changes through psychoactive drugs. Drugs are an external mechanism for making change within you and they limit important parts of your consciousness that won't be able to develop within you as they do when you climb the ladder of changes yourself.

To make changes inside, you have to change how you function, and that allows you to keep more of your daily conscious state within the expanded state. I'm not saying this to harsh your mellow but it's something that I think is true particularly for people like me who want to experience change in every part of their life through their own efforts. I'm not saying drugs are evil or anything like that, but I think they could keep you from climbing the ladder of personal evolution that exists within you through inner methods.

I am talking here through the lens of some personal experiences and not just old biases. My methods offer an alternative to achieving those states without the need for a chemical kick. They are slower and require more work and effort, but they also stay with you. They go where you go.

Achieving expanded states of consciousness will absolutely blow your mind, especially when you can achieve them anywhere, even if you're stuck in traffic or sitting on a plane. And, when you create them inside yourself, you can also turn them off at will. It is a lovely skill set for changing how you experience the life you are living right now, and it will also change how you show up in your life. It will open up a lot more of your potential and give you better capacity to work with your emotions.

TWENTY-SIX

THE FLOW MEDITATION

THIS MEDITATION IS WONDERFUL IN itself and as a center around which you can build a full meditation practice. It can bring you into a new brain state and into a new state of consciousness. I call it the flow meditation because it flows down inside your body. This meditation also works well to help you recover your energy in the middle of a stressful day or during a traumatic period in your life. It leads to a beautifully deep and relaxed state of consciousness.

1. Sit with your back straight and head up. Relax and take a deep breath.
2. Put your attention on the top of your head.
3. Move your attention to the space between your eyebrows and then straight back past your eyes into your brain.
4. Tell your nervous system that you want to focus on your pituitary gland and hypothalamus.
5. Leave your attention there until you feel satisfied that you got something done, up to a minute or two. There is no benefit in overdoing it.
6. Take a few moments to check on how you feel. Many people will think

this step is wasted time, but you are actively engaging more of you and engaging cross-connectivity in your brain.

Next, we will go a little further back in the brain to the pineal gland, closer to the brain stem but basically on the same line back. Again, remember the nervous system already knows precisely and without error where your brain stem is. You simply need to tune into it.

1. Sit the same position, feeling the suspension at the top of your head.
2. Move your attention to the spot between your eyebrows.
3. Move your attention straight back to the depth of your brain stem.
4. Tell your nervous system and subconscious mind that you want to center your attention on your pineal gland. Expect help and allow it to do the work. It's less important that your analytical mind is precise with this than it is that the feeling part of you shows you the way. Even if the space feels large or tiny don't question it. Just hold your attention there.
5. Hold your attention there until you feel satisfied or maybe even stimulated.
6. Observe how you feel. How does your body feel? How does your mind seem to you now?

How do you feel emotionally?

Note: At the end of each section I ask, "How do you feel emotionally?" The question could be asked in any section of the Activating Methods. They add a little extra perspective and suggestions for how to experience a sense of quality rather than simply following specific instructions.

Finally, we will do a set here that includes the pineal, pituitary, and hypothalamus together. There is an impressive feeling and change in state when they are accessed in conjunction.

1. Sit as above, paying attention to the crown of the head.

2. Move your attention down to the space between your eyebrows.
3. Lead your attention back to the last two centers, where we used the pituitary, hypothalamus, and pineal.
4. Tell your nervous system and subconscious mind what structures you want to work with.
5. Focus on these structures together and feel the connection between them—just a nice and easy connection with attention.
6. Hold your attention on these structures and their connection for a minute or two.
7. Check in on how you feel. Pay special attention to your brain state. How does your mind and consciousness seem to you now?

Please spend a little time working on these individually for a little while so you aren't overwhelmed when you put them together. They require practice to learn the position and the order of each without much thought. Eventually the exercises will begin to do themselves as you "watch yourself" doing them, but that kind of experience takes time, correct practice, and loads of attention to get to. It is extraordinary and beautiful when you do.

To get the most out of these methods you'll need to do them regularly, I would say at least every three days and preferably every day at this stage. Later, as you learn to put these all together, you can figure out how to pace yourself by how you feel. But for now, you need to get good enough with these to get the feeling you need to direct you to the next step.

All that being said, if you feel like you should stop, then stop. You will have to regulate yourself. All this inner work is really an inner-directed path. Only you know what is going on inside.

TWENTY-SEVEN

IMPORTANCE AND VALUE OF THE ACTIVATING METHODS

I'VE HAD A DIFFICULT TIME trying to express the importance of these methods. Some of this is, of course, a failure in my ability to communicate and to reframe complex ideas in a way people can understand. Some of it is my failure to understand why people don't see the same value in working with their mind, emotions, and body as I do. And some of it also has to do with some of the crazy experiences that I've had.

I actually know what it's like to be chained to a wall in a basement and not know if I'll ever get out. Because it is so extreme, that type of experience truly shows you who you are. It shows you what you have going on inside. But what a horrible teaching mechanism. There has to be a better way, and I think the methods I have created show you to yourself quite well. In some ways I'm trying to document my experiences with this because I think it'll be interesting and hopefully it will help me get the message across to more people.

Next to surviving, I think working on yourself on the inside is the single most important endeavor that a human can undertake. It's ultimately more important even than health because it can help restore your health, but you do need to be able to do the methods, so there are some base-level requirements of health to start with. However, if you can read and understand this, you are already capable of doing some of them.

One of my main purposes in this book is to try to make clear the value this kind of work has for you here and now. I have spent a fair amount of effort throughout this book to try to elucidate this idea. I am hoping by now you are starting to feel the truth of those words.

If you are trying to solve some health problems, these methods will help. If you are trying to make more money, these methods will help you think more clearly and regulate your emotions better. That will translate to a better ability to produce in work or business settings.

If you are lonely, you may be able to cut down the feeling by generating new brain states and activating what I believe is a response in your oxytocin through meditative states (I do this all the time, it's definitely possible). If you want to experience new states of consciousness, these methods will help.

If you want to sleep better, these methods can help. If you want to have a better time in your life, these methods can help you retrain yourself to feel pleasure and positive emotions (I've used them to do this). Being able to impact your own inner environment in a systematic and repeatable way, as far as I can tell, helps everything.

That might make the methods sound like a magic pill or snake oil. And fair enough, if you study advertising for even a few minutes you'll see lots of wild exaggeration. But I have no pills or oil to sell you. My methods require work. They require persistent practice. They require you to be willing to change and become something new. They require some small steps into the unknown. And they require you to buy, borrow, or check out a book or watch some videos online or come to a class. I can't think of a more productive thing to do.

Most people value things at a level similar to what they cost. Something that seems easy and free usually won't be seen as valuable. That's interesting. People will value a relationship that is hard because they had to fight for it more than a relationship that went so well it felt easy. We humans are funny creatures.

I can't price this work for what it is worth because of the high value I place on it myself. But fortunately, a candle doesn't diminish by lighting another candle. And so, I put it out there to give people who might value it a chance to find it and use it.

What I can't convey is its financial value. The price is you being willing to do the work yourself. All I can do is lead the way and give you some methods. Essentially, the value must be felt by the heart and intuition of anyone who pursues these powerful methods and the possibilities they hold. If you value them, I hope you will support me and my work to put them out there for more people to find and use.

I hope some of you will join me on the journey.

TWENTY-EIGHT

THE VITAL BRAIN METHOD

RECENTLY ONE OF MY GERMAN friends came up to me with a worried look in her eyes.

"Are you sure you want to teach these from America?" she said.

She said she thinks what I am doing with this work will make a substantial change in many people's lives and that had her concerned.

"Won't you be in danger of people coming after you for helping people heal without the use of drugs?" she said. "Aren't you nervous about the drug companies coming after you for cutting their profits?"

Then she proposed an idea: "Why don't you move to Germany? We could get married, and you could teach from Europe rather than from the U.S."

I was genuinely stunned. She'd just thrown a lot of hardcore information at me all at once. Honestly, I haven't had that many marriage proposals. I'm not exactly on the cover of *GQ* or *People* magazine's "Sexiest Man Alive." But I could tell she was genuinely worried about my safety because she thought my work was that groundbreaking.

I thought about everything she said. But I doubt that drug companies are worried about my brain-retraining methods making a dent in their profits. Still, her comments did reinforce for me how revolutionary this work might seem for some people. I realized that on some level I've become immune to the power of these methods, rendering me genuinely stunned by the reaction that people have to them. Including making someone want to marry me.

These methods might be extraordinarily useful for you and maybe a little bit revolutionary. Let's put together all the work we've been doing in this last major section of the book. I hope it works as well for you as it has for my German friend, who, sadly, had her marriage proposal turned down.

Here is where the rubber meets the road—the full method.

In this section we're going to put together everything we've learned to make the most use of all the parts in a comprehensive, synergistic method. In my view, we want to be as efficient as possible to get the biggest bang for our buck during our work.

If you are missing any of the structures we are working on with these methods—you've had your thyroid removed, for instance— just work where it was as if it were still there. Your body still has the map and the understanding of the machinery that was there.

I'm going to suggest two different versions that work well for slightly different things. The first version seems to give the greatest overall effect, specifically in generating health. The second version works a little better when you need energy and vitality as a pick-me-up. The first might be preferable before bed and the second earlier in the day or if you get tired in the afternoon.

If your main goal is to achieve expanded states, I would spend more time on the second one, but both will work. If you're feeling good and in good health and interested in getting the biggest change in state, I would try running the second version three times through.

The thing I wouldn't do, however, is to change the order of the Activating Methods or the order of the deep dive meditation. Those are built to create a specific effect on you and your system. You won't get the same effect if you change the order—at least at this point.

There are some interesting patterns we will get into later but there is a lot more for me to teach you before we start playing with activating patterns for effect. To do them you'll need to have mastered these and mastered the other base Activating Methods.

The main difference between the two versions that I will present here is that the first one starts with breathing exercises to get oxygen into the body to drive into the Activating Methods. Then we pull everything together with the meditations.

In the second version we'll do the meditations first to create a change in state, then we'll do the Activating Methods, and finally end with breathing, which will help oxygenate and energize your system to get you going for whatever you will do next. You might prefer one or the other or to alternate. Do whatever feels best to you.

Here's how you put this all together.

Start with the breathing exercises in this order:

1. Charging breath
2. Push breath
3. Layering breath

Then move onto the Activating Methods.

These are done in successive order, holding each area for up to three breaths. Then you move on to the next area. We want to create an effect by doing them in a particular order at a particular pace, at least at the beginning.

1. Sacral plexus
2. Spine
3. Heart
4. Brain stem
5. Limbic
6. Occipital
7. Parietal
8. Temporal
9. Frontal
10. Pituitary/Hypothalamus
11. Pineal
12. Pituitary/Hypothalamus and Pineal

Stacking the activating produces a powerful effect; it's absolutely incredible to experience. After a while, you'll get good enough at these methods that you won't have to think about them much and they will become easy and pleasurable to do.

Start by taking a few deep breaths, sitting up straight, and feeling suspended from above. Move your attention to each area one after another. At each area, hold for up to five full breaths (I often use three). Then move to the next area, until you finish the whole set.

You could stop there and just enjoy the feeling. I sometimes do. But the meditations at the end really tie things together and amplify the effect substantially. Play with it and see what you like and what feels good.

Then move on to the meditations in this order:

1. Meditation on glands and sense organs
2. Meditation on joints
3. Meninges meditation

Let's walk through this:

1. Take a moment to relax. Get yourself in the moment and then get into your body. Feel your body with your attention and consciousness.
2. Take in a deep, quick breath, like you are sucking in extra oxygen.
3. Pull that air up toward your lungs and into your brain. Your abdomen will expand during the in breath. Then you will gently push your abdomen in and feel your breath go up your torso and into your brain. This is a feeling exercise as much as a breathing exercise. You are encouraging a change in your system even though you aren't actually pushing oxygen into your brain.
4. Don't push out as much air as you took in. Just a simple exhalation to allow the gases in the air to change.
5. Repeat 30 times.
6. On the last breath, hold the breath gently, in and up as if the air is fueling your brain directly.
7. Let it out when it feels like you are just about to really need a breath. Don't force the hold but let it last for a while.
8. Lie on your back comfortably with your hands on your stomach.
9. Take in a quick deep breath and try to fill your stomach and then your chest with air. This inhalation should be quick and energetic, up to five or six seconds. This whole breath is meant to be done rather energetically.
10. Then take that air and push it into your arms and legs, leading it with your mind but also by contracting the muscles in your torso.
11. Push the exhalation out of your mouth and nose at the same time as pushing the air to your arms and legs and down to your hands and feet.
12. While doing the push, contract your belly into your spine and then push up the belly and diaphragm toward the head, creating a light

vacuum contraction. This will help push out the arms and legs but will also help stimulate the vagus nerve.

13. The vacuuming in the preceding breath will stimulate the next breath into a nice in and out cadence as you practice this breathing exercise.
14. Ten breaths in and out seem to be ideal to get something powerful done without stressing and straining yourself.
15. When you finish your breathing sequence, take a few minutes to check in on how you feel.
16. Find somewhere comfortable to sit, roll your hips forward, make your spine straight without force or tension, feel like your head is suspended from the ceiling.
17. Take an in breath, and "feel" the air go up your spine.
18. Contract the bottom of your pelvis in the space between your genitals and your anus, the perineum. This is just a very light contraction. Just enough to say you did it and no more than that.
19. During the same breath and after step 3, try to contract the space on the front of your sacrum and the front side of the back of your pelvis as well as the front side of the vertebrae of your lower back, the lumbar spine.
20. Contract the area of your solar plexus toward your spine and try to get some of that contraction on the front side of the spine opposite the solar plexus.
21. Feel a contraction on the upper third of the chest bone (sternum) right above the thymus, along with a contraction on the front of the spine directly opposite and a little above the thymus near the C7, T1, and T2 vertebrae.
22. Move on to the throat. Here we want to create a light contraction right at the midpoint as well as a very very light contraction on the upper two vertebrae and lowest part of the back of the skull. This will cover

THE VITAL BRAIN METHOD

the thyroid and the junction of your spine and skull.

23. This will bring our breath up to the brain and the top of the head. We want to hold our breath for just a comfortable amount of time when our attention reaches this area. Just enjoy the feeling of having lifted the breath and energy up to your brain and the top area of your head.

24. Exhale easily and without rushing. Start the same sequence with the next inhale.

Step 1

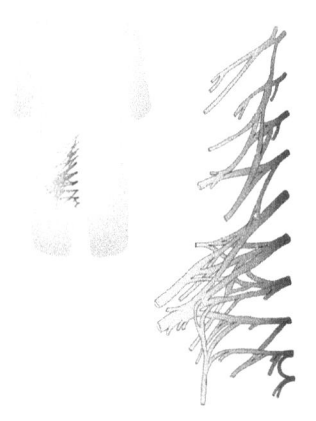

Lumbosacral nerve plexus

We will start with the lumbosacral nerve plexus, a web of nerves in the lumbar and sacral region of the body. It sits on the front side of your lower back, running through the front of your pelvis, down into your legs.

Direct your attention to this nerve plexus and try to reconnect to the part of you that can feel it. This is all about putting your attention there and holding it for a few moments until it feels that your attention "activated" it. Leave it there for a few moments.

Step 2 - The spine

In this step we will be using the entirety of the spine from the neck down to the sacrum. We will not only use the bone but also everything inside, including the meninges, the cerebral spinal fluid, and the spinal cord. Move your attention here and hold it for a few moments.

Step 3 - The heart

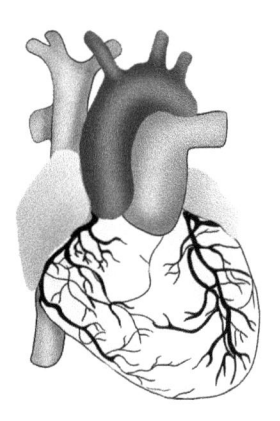

Heart

The heart is in your upper chest a little bit left of the centerline just off the sternum and protected by the ribs. It pumps your blood and is integral to getting oxygen into the blood from the lungs. What people often don't know is that your heart also has a large collection of sensory dendrites, generally around 40,000, which act like a small brain.

The brain stem

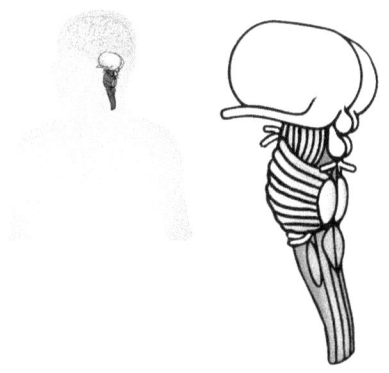

Brain stem

Now we will be working with the base of your brain where it meets your spinal cord. The brain stem is the posterior part of the brain that connects the cerebrum with the spinal cord. If you think of working where the top of your spine meets the base of your skull inside the upper vertebrae and the tissue that goes through the hole at the bottom of your skull, you'll be in the right area for this work.

The limbic brain

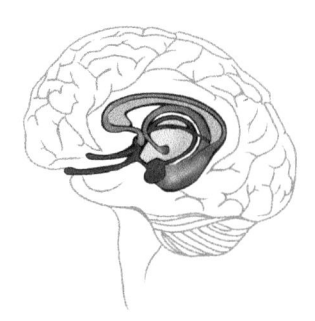

Limbic system

You will find this structure right above the brain stem. So, take your attention from where it was and move it slightly upward, so it sits right above the brain stem, very deep in your brain.

The occipital lobe

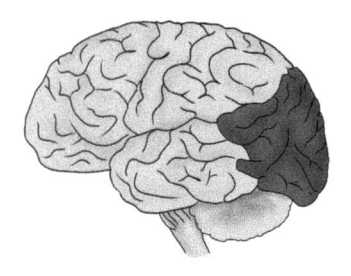

Occipital lobe

Move your attention to the part of your brain that is just inside the back of your skull and above the spine. Try to get your attention about an inch inside the skull. Feel your way to it. Hold your attention there for a few moments.

The parietal lobes

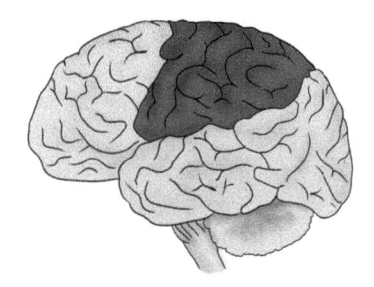

Parietal lobe

Gently move your attention to the parietal lobes. These sit right under the top of your skull from the top of the occipital lobe to the back of the frontal lobe, which sits right behind your forehead.

The temporal lobes

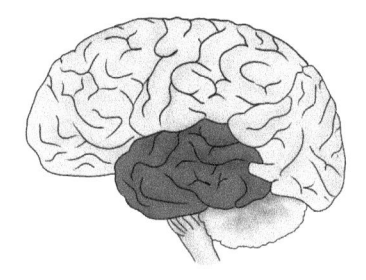

Temporal lobe

Your temporal lobes begin behind your temples and then run behind your ears until they meet your occipital lobe in the back. It's a larger area than you might think. Draw your attention to the occipital lobe. Hold your attention in this area for a few moments.

The frontal lobe

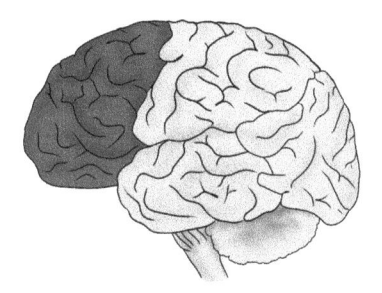

Frontal lobe

Move your attention to the space right behind your frontal bone, your forehead. Go one to two inches behind the bone. Don't worry about being super specific.

The pituitary gland and hypothalamus

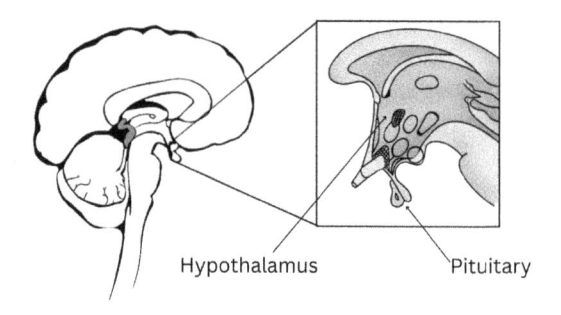

Hypothalamus — Pituitary

Pituitary & hypothalamus

Move your attention to the space between your eyebrows and then straight back past your eyes into your brain. Tell your nervous system that you want to focus on your pituitary gland and hypothalamus.

The pineal gland

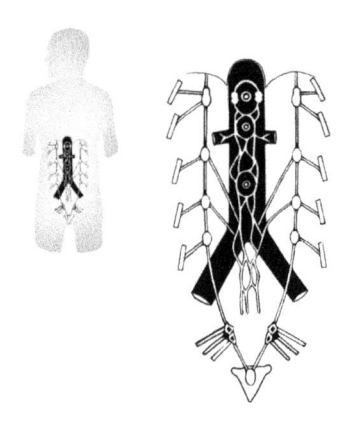

Celiac plexus

Next, we will go a little further back, closer to the brain stem but basically on the same line back. Move your attention straight back until you get close to the depth of your brain stem. Tell your nervous system and subconscious mind that you want to center your attention on your pineal gland. Hold your attention there until you feel satisfied.

The pineal and pituitary/hypothalamus together.

1. Lead your attention back to the last two centers we used for the pituitary/hypothalamus and the pineal.
2. Tell your nervous system and subconscious mind what structures you want to work with.
3. Focus on these structures together and feel the connection between them—just a nice and easy connection with attention.
4. Hold your attention on these structures and their connection for a few moments.

Meditation Section

1. Sit up straight, roll your hips slightly forward, lift the top of your head toward the sky, and feel it lightly held up at the crown of your head.
2. Take a few minutes to let everything relax and let your breathing become slow and deep.

Don't force any of this.

3. Put your attention on the crown of your head, the very top where the soft spot was when you were a baby. Gently hold that attention for up to a minute.
4. Draw your attention down the center of your forehead to the space between your eyebrows. Just draw a line there with your attention, feeling as the line goes from point to point in a relaxed, slow, and deliberate way.

5. Draw your attention from the point between your eyebrows toward the back of your head until your attention gets to your pituitary gland.

6. Run your attention through the gland to activate and relax it. Activation here just means to wake it up through your attention to it. Your nervous system already knows where it is and how to reach it. You just need to reconnect to what is already known subconsciously. Intellectualizing and getting lost in your memory are the opposite of what we want to accomplish here. We actually want to give the intellect a break to slow down, and we want to free ourselves from the demands of memory.

7. Now that we have activated the pituitary gland, we will move farther toward the back of the head to reach the pineal gland.

8. Lead your attention and mind to the pineal gland and activate it by running your attention through it.

9. Draw your attention forward to the space between your eyes. Lead it down over your nose, mouth, and chin to reach the front of your neck. Here we will find the thyroid gland, which is in front of the tubes in your throat—roughly in the middle.

10. 10) Run your attention through the thyroid until you feel satisfied that you did it thoroughly. Again, don't force this. There are no grades, no one is watching, so this is your gig. Make it feel good and work for you. This won't work if you strain.

11. Draw your attention from the center of your throat down to the point where your collarbones meet in the center. Here you'll find the top of the sternum and at the top third of the sternum you'll find the thymus gland.

12. Lead your attention through your thymus to wake up and activate this gland. Your mind and attention are way more powerful than you might think. Putting your attention on different aspects of yourself and your physical body produces interesting effects in you, your emotions, your

mind, and ultimately your consciousness. Most people never experience this because they've always put almost all their attention on the outside world, trying to control that. They have missed the power of working inside themselves.

13. After working with the thymus in a satisfying way, take your attention further down your torso to the lower side of your sternum where there is no bone. Then lead your attention back toward your spine until you almost reach it. Here you will find the celiac plexus.

14. Will your mind and attention through the celiac plexus until you have satisfyingly created the activation you are looking for or at least until you feel comfortable to move on. Adequate is good enough, perfectionism will block what you are trying to create here.

15. Now draw your attention down from the celiac plexus straight toward your hips until you reach your kidneys, on top of which you will find your adrenal glands.

16. Bisect your attention onto both adrenal glands at the same time and again run your attention through the glands until you feel satisfied, like you've gotten something done. Keep it nice and easy. Nothing serious is going on here, you're just getting something useful to happen inside.

17. Move your attention further down into your pelvis until you reach your testes or ovaries. If you have had your ovaries removed, imagine where they were and do this in your imagination. With as much ease and relaxation as possible, run your attention through your ovaries or testicles until you feel like you're done. No strain, no seriousness, no pain, no grades, no perfectionism, no performing—just play with it. Play with all of these.

18. Now sit and relax, try not to jump up and rush out unless you absolutely have to. It's good to take a few minutes to let your nervous system absorb and reflect the changes you've just made so they can become permanent.

1. Sit somewhere comfortable. Feel like the top of your head is being held up by a string suspended from the ceiling, gently lifting your entire spine.
2. Aim your attention toward your shoulders, both sides at once. Run your attention through each shoulder and into the joint.
3. Now move your attention down to your elbows and the joint in the center of the structures until it feels like you are done. Don't force, don't try to do it perfectly, don't get lost in an image of the anatomical structure. Play with it, have some fun with it, and try to feel everything in the joint as you run your mind to the center.
4. Move onto your wrists. Going outside to inside will draw your attention into the center of your wrists. It's interesting to use your attention to quiet your mind and help it relearn how to feel at a deeper level. This will change your use of attention and ultimately your consciousness.
5. Now, go through your hands, wrist side down, toward the fingers, paying special attention to each of the knuckles. Take your time going through the hands, there's a lot going on there and a lot of joints to work through. Have some fun with it. It might be helpful at first to go finger by finger, but later it will be faster to do them all collectively. Try to be thorough and not to miss anything. Feel it all.
6. Move your attention to the hip joints and playfully move your attention from the outside to inside the joint, going superficially to deep. These joints are a little bigger so there's more for your mind to play with to get a good feeling from what you were doing.
7. Draw your attention to the knees, going from the outside to the inside as deep into the knee as you can. When it feels complete, you're done. Don't let your analytical judgment take over your feeling sense, because that will make you lose the effect that we're

trying to create with these meditative processes.

8. Move down to your ankles. Make sure to feel the bones (malleoli) on either side. Start there and move your way deep into the joints, playfully experiencing them with your attention until you reach the centers of the ankle. Let go of everything else as you do it. Keep your attention and mind here, away from the future or the past or anything you feel like you have to get done right this second. Nothing else exists at this moment but your ankles.

9. Finally, we get to the feet. Move your attention down from the ankles, through your heels, and into the rest of your feet, feeling as much of them as you can. Pay special attention as you finally get down into the joints, working your attention playfully to the tips of your toes and toenails. Make it fun, make it playful, nothing serious is going on here, it's just something that's useful for every part of you.

10. Now take a few minutes to check how you feel. Putting your attention on how you feel can help keep your mind calm until you're ready to move back into your day and crush your life.

The Meninges Meditation

1. Sit up straight.
2. On your next inhale, run your breath from your tailbone up around your skull on the inside of the bone. Get used to the inhale moving up your spine.
3. On the exhale, run your breath from around your brain under the skull bones down the inside of the spine to your tailbone.
4. Inhale up and exhale down. Practice a few rounds of this until you get the hang of it.
5. Once you get the hang of it, put your attention on the dura mater and

run your breath along this tissue from tailbone to around your brain.
6. Run your breath down the same tissue from around your brain down your spine to the tailbone.
7. Move on to the arachnoid mater, the middle layer of the meninges. On the in breath, move up the middle layer. Move down the middle layer on the out breath.
8. Moving down to the deepest layer of the meninges, the pia mater, move up the deepest layer on the in breath and move down on the out breath.
9. Once you finish this, go back to the outside layer and start the process again, outside to inside.
10. Repeat this cycle until you feel like you've gotten something done. This can be anywhere from a few minutes to hours depending on how you feel.

Alternate method:

1. Meditation on glands and sense organs
2. Meditation on joints
3. Meninges meditation

Activating Methods

1. Sacral plexus
2. Spine
3. Heart
4. Brain stem
5. Limbic
6. Occipital
7. Parietal
8. Temporal

9. Frontal
10. Pituitary/Hypothalamus
11. Pineal
12. Pituitary/Hypothalamus and Pineal

Breathing Methods

1. Charging breath
2. Push breath
3. Layering breath

TWENTY-NINE

FINAL THOUGHTS

THANK YOU FOR READING MY book and giving it your precious time and attention. It's my hope that I shared something extraordinarily valuable with you here. These methods changed my life in such a profound way, and I hope they will do the same for you. Many people, myself included, feel stuck in their lives and within themselves. But there are options and possibilities, so don't stop trying to make your life experience and your life better! I did it and so can you!

Remember, the results will come with practice and depth of ability to apply them to your own life. I'm firmly of the opinion that anyone can do these methods successfully with practice, belief in the methods, and belief in your own ability to get something done.

Now that you have read this book, I encourage you to return time and time again and try these methods yourself. Try to keep in mind what you wanted to get out of this book: How do you think the information in this book could help you, and how do you see yourself using it? What is the biggest personal pain point in your life? I also encourage you to allow your analytical mind to have a nap. Let it relax and allow the rest of you to do the work. This will give you the freedom to step out of the box.

If you stay in the familiar and don't venture beyond your comfort zone, you will miss many of the possible benefits here. If your analytical mind is running your attention, you'll never really be able to access the part of your mind involved in feeling and intuition. Now is the time to take back more of your potential! Play with this, have fun, and experience it. That's where the magic lies. People are told way too often that they can't do things or aren't capable. Watch out for those people who tell you what you can or cannot do. Often, they know you can do it and watching you succeed would make them jealous. This has nothing to do with you. They are using it as a power game to activate their own serotonin and maintain some social dominance.

No one, not even you, knows what you are capable of. You probably haven't ever pushed yourself to half of what you might be capable of, and you probably haven't been pushed so hard into a corner that the lion within you roars.

You've got this. You can do this. You matter!

Until next time, stay vital.

THIRTY

GLOSSARY

ADRENAL GLANDS – Endocrine glands that produce a variety of hormones including adrenaline.

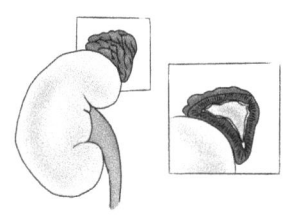

Adrenal gland

ALPHA BRAIN WAVE – Medium frequency waves that are commonly observed when people feel relaxed and the brain in in an idle state.

ARACHNOID MATER MENINGES – The middle layer located underneath the dura mater. It consists of connective tissue, is avascular and does not receive any innervation.

BETA BRAIN WAVE – High frequency low amplitude waves that are commonly observed while awake and in engaged in mental activities.

BRAIN STEM – The distal part of the brain that is made up of the midbrain, pons, and medulla oblongata. It connects the cerebrum with the spinal cord.

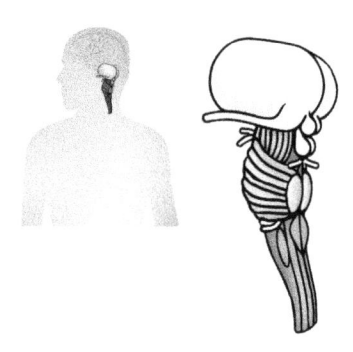

Brain stem

CELIAC PLEXUS – A nerve plexus that is situated in the abdomen behind the stomach.

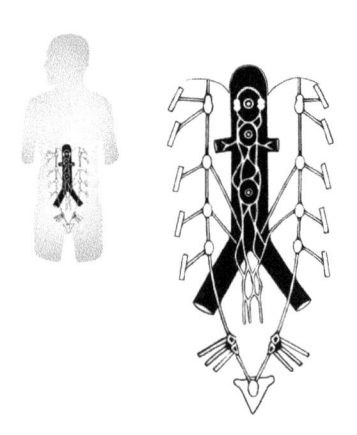

Celiac plexus

DELTA BRAIN WAVE – High amplitude brain wave commonly observed with deep sleep. It is the slowest brain wave with the highest amplitude.

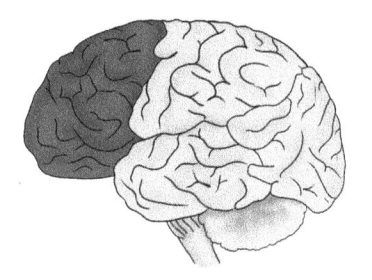

Frontal lobe

DURA MATER MENINGES – The outermost layer located directly underneath the bones of the skull. It is thick, tough and inextensible.

FRONTAL LOBE – The part of the brain responsible for processing behavior, learning, personality and voluntary movement.

GAMMA BRAIN WAVE – The highest frequency of all brain waves. They are associated with high levels of thought and focus.

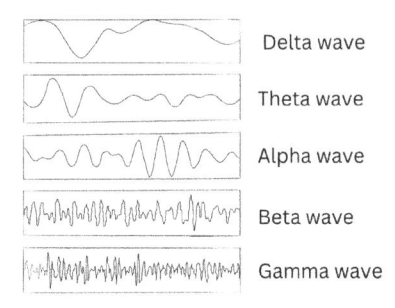

Delta wave
Theta wave
Alpha wave
Beta wave
Gamma wave

Brain waves

HEART – The muscle that pumps blood received from veins into arteries throughout the body.

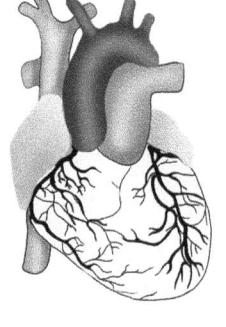

Heart

HYPOTHALAMUS – A region of the forebrain below the thalamus which coordinates both the autonomic nervous system and the activity of the pituitary.

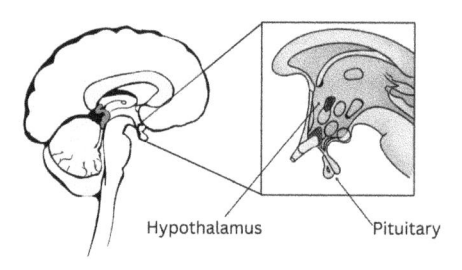

Pituitary & hypothalamus

LIMBIC SYSTEM – A set of brain structures located on both sides of the thalamus. It governs emotions, motivation, olfaction, and behavior. It is also involved in the formation of long-term memory.

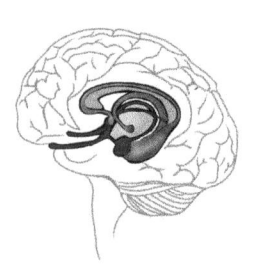

Limbic system

LUMBOSACRAL NERVE PLEXUS – A network of nerves that supplies the lower limb and pelvic girdle.

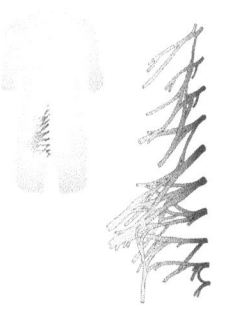

Lumbosacral nerve plexus

OCCIPITAL LOBE – The part of the brain responsible for processing visual information.

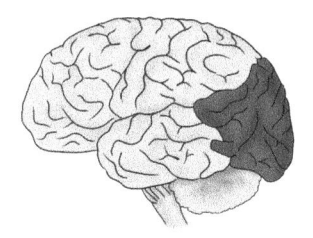

Occipital lobe

OVARIES – A female reproductive organ in which ova and eggs are produced.

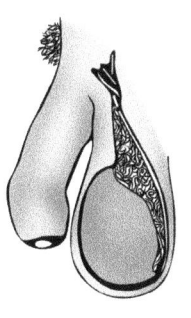

Testes

PARIETAL LOBE – The part of the brain responsible for processing sensory information received from touch, taste, and temperature. It also plays a role in navigation, control and spatial awareness.

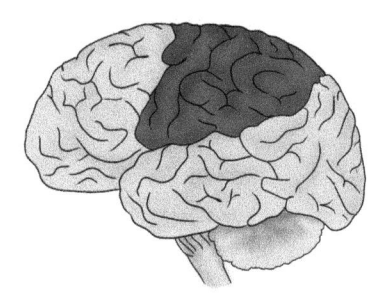

Parietal lobe

PIA MATER MENINGES – The innermost layer, it closely covers the brain. It acts as a barrier and helps in the production of cerebrospinal fluid.

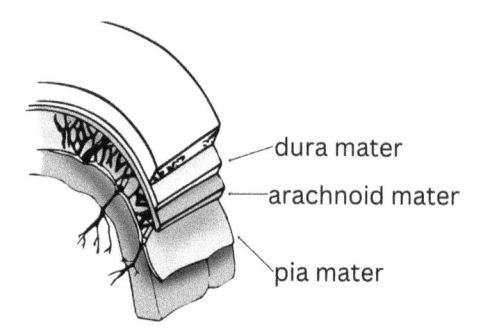

Meninges

PINEAL GLAND – A small endocrine gland in the brain. The pineal gland produces melatonin.

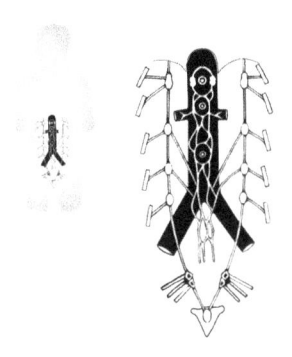

Celiac plexus

PITUITARY GLAND – A small pea-sized endocrine gland located at the base of the brain. It produces hormones that affect many body functions.

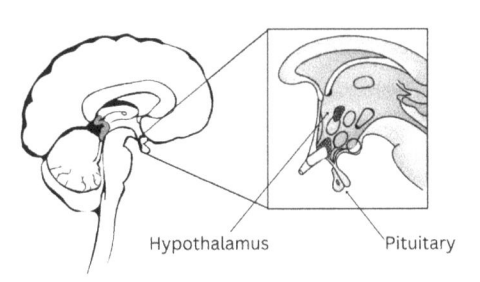

Hypothalamus   Pituitary

Pituitary & hypothalamus

TEMPORAL LOBE – The part of the brain responsible for processing information from sensory input, especially hearing and language.

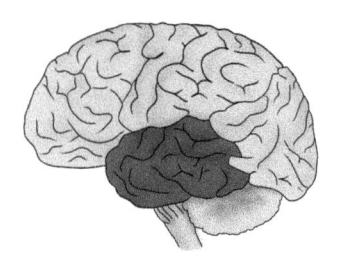

Temporal lobe

TESTES – An organ which produces spermatozoa (male reproductive cells.)

THETA BRAIN WAVE – A type of neural oscillation, that underlies various aspects of cognition and behavior such as learning and memory. They occur when sleeping or dreaming but not in deep sleep.

THYMUS – An organ that is part of the lymphatic system, in which Lymphocytes grow and multiply.

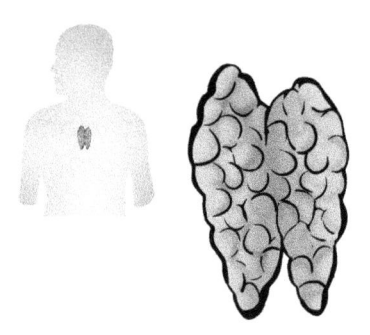

Thymus

ENDNOTES

1 Lauren Silva, "What Is Somatic Therapy?" *Forbes Health*, last modified June 14, 2023, https://www.forbes.com/health/mind/somatic-therapy/

2 "Nytality Method," *Nytality Method*, accessed June 30, 2023, https://www.nytality.com/.

3 "Dr. Foojan Zeine," Dr. Foojan Zeine, accessed June 30, 2023, https://foojanzeine.com/.

4 "Wim Hof Method," Wim Hof Method, accessed June 30, 2023, https://www.wimhofmethod.com/breathing-exercises.

5 "Pineal Gland," Cleveland Clinic, accessed June 30, 2023, https://my.clevelandclinic.org/health/body/23334-pineal-gland.

6 Ned Herrmann, "What Is the Function of the Various Brainwaves?", Scientific American, last modified December 22, 1997, https://www.scientificamerican.com/article/what-is-the-function-of-t-1997-12-22/.

7 "Oxytocin," Cleveland Clinic, last modified March 27, 2022, https://my.clevelandclinic.org/health/articles/22618-oxytocin.

8 Anna Hernández, "Lumbosacral Plexus," Osmosis, accessed June 30, 2023, https://www.osmosis.org/answers/lumbosacral-plexus.

9 Hayden Basinger and Jeffrey P. Hogg, "Neuroanatomy, Brainstem," National Library of Medicine, last modified July 6, 2022, https://www.ncbi.nlm.nih.gov/books/NBK544297/.

10 V. Rajmohand and E. Mohandas, "The Limbic System," *Indian Journal of Psychiatry* 49, no. 2 (2007): 132-39, doi: 10.4103/0019-5545.33264.

11 "Occipital Lobe," Cleveland Clinic, last modified December 22, 2022, https://my.clevelandclinic.org/health/body/24498-occipital-lobe.

12 "Parietal Lobe," Cleveland Clinic, last modified January 8, 2023, https://my.clevelandclinic.org/health/body/24628-parietal-lobe.

13 "Temporal Lobe," Cleveland Clinic, last modified January 8, 2023, https://my.clevelandclinic.org/health/body/16799-temporal-lobe.

14 "Frontal Lobe," Cleveland Clinic, last modified December 5, 2022, https://my.clevelandclinic.org/health/body/24501-frontal-lobe.

15 Matt Smith, "What Is Cerebrospinal Fluid?", WebMD, last modified May 4, 2023, https://www.webmd.com/brain/cerebrospinal-fluid-facts.

16 "Meninges," Cleveland Clinic, last modified January 11, 2022, https://my.clevelandclinic.org/health/articles/22266-meninges.

17 "Meninges," Cleveland Clinic.

18 "The Pituitary Gland," Cleveland Clinic, last modified April 4, 2022, https://my.clevelandclinic.org/health/body/21459-pituitary-gland.

19 "Hypothalamus," Cleveland Clinic, last modified March 16, 2022, https://my.clevelandclinic.org/health/articles/22566-hypothalamus.

20 "Pineal Gland," Cleveland Clinic, last modified June 22, 2022, https://my.clevelandclinic.org/health/body/23334-pineal-gland.

Milton Keynes UK
Ingram Content Group UK Ltd.
UKHW030811130224
437765UK00014B/565